Osteoporosis Diet Cookbook Recipes For Seniors

Delicious and Nutritious Science-Based and
Calcium Fortified Recipes for Men and
Women with Osteoporosis

Samantha Bax

Osteoporosis Diet Cookbook Recipes for Seniors
Samantha Bax

Copyright 2023 © Prose Books LLC

ISBN: 978-1-963160-10-9

All rights reserved.

No portion of this book may be reproduced without written permission from the publisher or author except as permitted by U.S. copyright law.

This publication is designed to provide accurate and authoritative information regarding the subject matter covered. It is sold with the understanding that neither the author nor the publisher is engaged in rendering legal, investment, accounting, or other professional services.

While the publisher and author have used their best efforts in preparing this book, they make no representations or warranties with respect to the accuracy or completeness of the contents of this book and specifically disclaim any implied warranties of merchantability or fitness for a particular purpose. Sales representatives or written sales materials may create or extend no warranty.

The advice and strategies contained herein may not be suitable for your situation. You should consult with a professional when appropriate. Neither the publisher nor the author shall be liable for any loss of profit or other commercial damages, including but not limited to special, incidental, consequential, personal, or other damages.

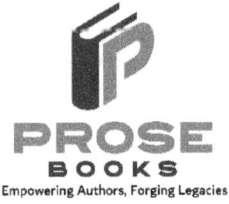

Prose Books
Prose Books LLC
Merrimack, NH 03054 USA
email: info@prosebooks.com

Table of Contents

Table of Contents iii
Chapter 1: Introduction 1
   Overview of Osteoporosis and Its Impact on Bone Health 1
Chapter 2: The Basics of Bone-Healthy Eating 3
   Developing a Strong Foundation for a Diet that Supports Healthy Bones 3
   Essential Nutrients for Optimal Bone Health and Their Food Sources 3
Chapter 3: Breakfast and Smoothie Recipes 6
   Recipe 1: Creamy Banana-Oat Breakfast Smoothie 7
   Recipe 2: Spinach and Feta Breakfast Quesadilla 8
   Recipe 3: Berry-Almond Greek Yogurt Parfait 9
   Recipe 4: Veggie and Cheese Omelet 10
   Recipe 5: Blueberry and Almond Chia Pudding 11
   Recipe 6: Quinoa and Spinach Breakfast Bowl 12
   Recipe 7: Whole-Grain Banana Pancakes 13
   Recipe 8: Avocado and Tomato Toast with Poached Eggs 14
   Recipe 9: Almond and Berry Breakfast Quinoa Bowl 15
   Recipe 10: Cinnamon Apple Overnight Oats 16
Chapter 4: Nourishing Soups and Salads - Savor the Flavors of Bone 17
   Recipe 11: Creamy Broccoli and Cheddar Soup 18
   Recipe 12: Spinach and Strawberry Salad with Poppy Seed Dressing 19
   Recipe 13: Lentil and Kale Soup 20
   Recipe 14: Grilled Chicken and Quinoa Salad 21
   Recipe 15: Butternut Squash and Kale Salad 22
   Recipe 16: Creamy Tomato Basil Soup 23
   Recipe 17: Chickpea and Spinach Salad with Tahini Dressing 24
   Recipe 18: Quinoa and Black Bean Soup 25
   Recipe 19: Arugula and Roasted Beet Salad 26
   Recipe 20: Sweet Potato and Quinoa Salad 27
Chapter 5: Wholesome Main Courses - Nourishing Your Bones with Every Bite 28
   Recipe 21: Baked Salmon with Lemon-Dill Sauce 29

- Recipe 22: Quinoa-Stuffed Bell Peppers 30
- Recipe 23: Spinach and Mushroom Stuffed Chicken Breast 31
- Recipe 24: Lentil and Vegetable Stir-Fry 32
- Recipe 25: Grilled Chicken and Vegetable Skewers with Yogurt-Herb Sauce 33
- Recipe 26: Eggplant Parmesan 34
- Recipe 27: Tofu and Broccoli Stir-Fry 35
- Recipe 28: Beef and Vegetable Stir-Fry 36
- Recipe 29: Chickpea and Spinach Curry 37
- Recipe 30: Quinoa and Black Bean Stuffed Bell Peppers 38

Chapter 6: Sides and Snacks for Strong Bones 39
- Recipe 31: Mango Salsa 40
- Recipe 32: Avocado and Tomato Bruschetta 41
- Recipe 33: Spinach and Artichoke Dip 42
- Recipe 34: Walnut and Cranberry Quinoa Salad 43
- Recipe 35: Guacamole with Veggie Sticks 44
- Recipe 36: Baked Sweet Potato Chips 45
- Recipe 37: Mixed Berry Smoothie Bowl 46
- Recipe 38: Quinoa Salad with Cranberries and Almonds 47
- Recipe 39: Carrot and Raisin Salad 48
- Recipe 40: Almond and Date Energy Bites 49

Chapter 7: Desserts and Treats - Satisfy Your Sweet Tooth with Bone 50
- Recipe 41: Creamy Berry Parfait 51
- Recipe 42: Chia Seed Pudding with Almonds and Dates 52
- Recipe 43: Frozen Banana Bites 53
- Recipe 44: Chocolate Avocado Mousse 54
- Recipe 45: Almond and Oat Cookies 55
- Recipe 46: Greek Yogurt and Honey Popsicles 56
- Recipe 47: Mango and Coconut Chia Popsicles 57
- Recipe 48: Berry and Yogurt Bark 58
- Recipe 49: Frozen Yogurt Banana Pops 59
- Recipe 50: Cinnamon Apple Crisp 60

Chapter 8: Meal Plans and Tips for Success 61

Sample Meal Plan 1: Balanced Diet 62
Sample Meal Plan 2: Vegetarian and Calcium-Rich 63
Sample Meal Plan 3: Vegan and Calcium-Focused 64
Sample Meal Plan 4: Mediterranean Diet for Bone Health 65
Sample Meal Plan 5: Plant-Based and Calcium-Rich 66
Sample Meal Plan 6: Low-Carb and Bone-Healthy 67
Chapter 9: Bonus Recipes – Culinary Delights for Extraordinary Bone Health 68
    Recipe 51: Greek Yogurt Pancakes..69
    Recipe 52: Quinoa Salad with Roasted Vegetables............................70
    Recipe 53: Lemon Herb Grilled Chicken 71
    Recipe 54: Roasted Chickpeas Snack...72
    Recipe 55: Berry and Almond Parfait 73
    Recipe 56: Mediterranean Hummus Wrap 74
    Recipe 57: Lemon Garlic Shrimp and Asparagus 75
    Recipe 58: Mixed Berry Chia Pudding...76
    Recipe 59: Avocado Chocolate Mousse..77
    Recipe 60: Sweet Potato and Black Bean Breakfast Burrito 78
Chapter 10: Conclusion..79
Appendix: Additional Resources 81
About The Author 84
Other Books by Samantha Bax 86
Thank You..89
FREE Meal-Planner 90

Osteoporosis Diet Cookbook Recipes for Seniors - Samantha Bax

Chapter 1: Introduction

Overview of Osteoporosis and Its Impact on Bone Health

Osteoporosis is a bone condition characterized by bone mass, deterioration of bone tissue, and an increased risk of fractures. It affects several people, especially women who are over 50 years old. This chapter will provide an overview of osteoporosis and its impact on bone health. We will emphasize the importance of maintaining a diet to manage this condition effectively. Additionally, we will explore scientifically proven recipes enriched with calcium to help maintain and improve bone health.

Osteoporosis is often referred to as a "disease" because it progresses silently without displaying symptoms until a fracture occurs. The bones affected by osteoporosis weaken, making individuals more prone to fractures in the spine, hips, and wrists. These fractures can have consequences such as pain, disability, loss of independence, and even increased mortality rates.

The main cause of osteoporosis is an imbalance between bone formation and resorption, resulting in bone density loss over time. Several factors contribute to this imbalance, including age, genetic predisposition, hormonal changes, inadequate intake of calcium and vitamin D in the diet or through supplements leading a lifestyle or being physically inactive for periods, smoking tobacco products excessively, consuming alcohol regularly as well as certain medications that may increase the risk. Given the nature of osteoporosis and the contributing factors involved, taking a comprehensive approach to its management is crucial by giving special attention to diet and nutrition.

Maintaining bone health and managing osteoporosis require a balanced diet. Calcium, a mineral for bones, can be obtained from both sources and supplements. It's important to ensure calcium intake to support the formation of strong bones as they serve as a storage site for calcium in the body. Good sources of calcium include dairy products, leafy green vegetables, cereals, and calcium supplements. However, it's worth noting that calcium alone is not enough for bone health; other nutrients like vitamin D, magnesium, phosphorus, and vitamin K also play roles.

Vitamin D is essential for the absorption and utilization of calcium. It can be produced by the skin when exposed to sunlight or obtained from sources such as fatty fish, egg yolks, and fortified products. Magnesium and phosphorus are also minerals that greatly contribute to bone health by supporting the integrity of bones. Foods rich in magnesium include nuts, seeds, legumes, and whole grains, while dairy products, fish, meat, and nuts are sources of phosphorus.

Lastly, a team of experts has developed a science-based and calcium-fortified strategy for creating recipes to help individuals with osteoporosis adopt a diet promoting bones. These recipes include ingredients to ensure health benefits and a delightful culinary experience. By incorporating foods in calcium like dairy products, leafy greens, and fortified alternatives, these recipes offer a delicious way to get the essential nutrients. Moreover, they are carefully designed to maintain balance by providing amounts of vitamin D, magnesium, phosphorus, and vitamin K—all crucial for supporting bone health.

The science-based recipe approach also emphasizes the significance of patterns. It encourages the consumption of foods from groups, ensuring a well-rounded intake of macronutrients (carbohydrates, proteins, and fats) and micronutrients (vitamins and minerals). This approach discourages diets while promoting foods over processed or sugary options that may adversely affect bone health.

In summary, osteoporosis is a concern affecting bone health, increasing the risk of fractures, and reducing quality of life. Managing osteoporosis and maintaining bone health requires a diet rich in calcium, vitamin D, magnesium, phosphorus, and vitamin K.

Incorporating a calcium-enriched method into our recipes allows us to savor meals that fulfill our nutritional requirements. In the chapters, we will explore dietary suggestions, provide recipe illustrations, and offer practical advice to support your quest for robust and nourished bones.

Chapter 2: The Basics of Bone-Healthy Eating

Developing a Strong Foundation for a Diet that Supports Healthy Bones

Maintaining healthy bones while preventing conditions such as osteoporosis relies heavily on nutrition. This section will explore the basics of a bone diet, focusing on nutrients, food choices, and practical tips for meal planning and grocery shopping. By incorporating these strategies into your routine, you'll be well on your way to maintaining robust bones.

Essential Nutrients for Optimal Bone Health and Their Food Sources

To promote the growth and upkeep of bones, consuming a rounded diet that includes specific nutrients is crucial. Let's delve into four nutrients and the primary food sources associated with them.

Calcium: Calcium is the cornerstone of bone health by providing strength and density to prevent fractures and osteoporosis. Excellent dietary sources of calcium include dairy products like milk, cheese, and yogurt as fortified plant-based alternatives. Leafy greens like kale, broccoli, and bok choy are also rich in calcium. Additionally, certain fish like canned salmon or sardines (including their bones) offer a calcium boost.

Vitamin D: Vitamin D plays a role in facilitating calcium absorption within the body—an aspect of bone health. Sunlight exposure is the source of vitamin D; however, it can also be found in fish, like salmon and mackerel.

If you don't get the sun, including vitamin D-fortified foods like milk, orange juice, and cereals in your diet is beneficial.

Protein: This is important for building and repairing bones. It provides the components for developing bones and muscles. Good protein sources include meats, poultry, fish, legumes, nuts, and seeds. Ensuring you have various protein sources in your meals will help you get all the amino acids you need.

Magnesium: Magnesium plays a role in converting vitamin D into its form and maintaining proper bone density. Foods rich in magnesium include leafy vegetables, whole grains, nuts, seeds, and legumes. Incorporating these foods into your meals can help meet your magnesium needs.

Here are some practical tips to help with meal planning and grocery shopping for osteoporosis:

Create a meal plan that includes a variety of rich foods. Base your meals around calcium options like yogurt with fruit for breakfast or a green salad with salmon for lunch. Include meats or legumes as the component of your dinner to ensure sufficient protein intake.

To maintain healthy bones, it's important to incorporate a variety of colorful fruits and vegetables into your diet. Aim for five servings daily, including leafy greens, citrus fruits, berries, and cruciferous vegetables like broccoli and cauliflower.

When you go grocery shopping, take the time to read food labels carefully. Look for products fortified with calcium and vitamin D. However, be mindful of added sugars and sodium, as excessive amounts can impact your bone health.

If you follow a plant-based diet or are intolerant, explore plant-based alternatives fortified with calcium. Almond, soy, or oat milk can be options for you. Additionally, include plant-based protein sources such as tofu, tempeh, and legumes in your meals.

While it is always best to get your nutrients from foods, sometimes dietary supplements can help ensure you're getting calcium, vitamin D, and magnesium. It is recommended to consult with a healthcare before starting any supplements.

By incorporating these tips into your routine, you'll build a foundation for maintaining healthy bones and reducing the risk of osteoporosis. To sum up, it is important to have a diet to maintain healthy bones. This means including nutrients like calcium, vitamin D, protein, and magnesium in your meals.

By incorporating various foods from food groups and following tips, planning meals, and shopping for groceries, you can ensure that your bones get the nourishment they need to stay strong and resilient. This chapter will delve into the importance of activity and how it promotes bone health.

Chapter 3: Breakfast and Smoothie Recipes

Welcome to Chapter 3 of your "Osteoporosis Diet Cookbook." In this chapter, we'll explore the world of breakfasts and smoothies that promote healthy bones. Breakfast is often considered the day's meal, and for good reason. It provides the energy and nutrients needed to kickstart your day and support your well-being.

In this section, we've curated a collection of morning recipes that not only tantalize your taste buds but also prioritize your bone health. We understand that mornings can be hectic. That doesn't mean you have to compromise on nutrition. Whether you prefer a breakfast to satisfy you until lunch or a quick yet nutritious smoothie to grab on the go, we have something for everyone.

Our recipes incorporate ingredients in calcium sources of vitamin D and other essential nutrients known for their benefits in strengthening bones. You'll discover various flavors, textures, and ingredients that will make preparing and savoring your morning meals an experience.

From creamy and comforting bowls to vibrant smoothie creations packed with nutrients, these recipes will inspire you to start your day off. We've also included cooking tips and nutritional information so that you can choose what goes on your morning menu.

Whether savoring a relaxed morning meal at home or seeking a convenient smoothie to power through your day, turn to Chapter 3 as your trusted guide for breakfasts promoting strong bones. Here's to fueling your body with nourishing bites one at a time!

Recipe 1: Creamy Banana-Oat Breakfast Smoothie

Prep Time: 5 minutes - Cooking Time: 0 minutes - Number of Servings: 2

Ingredients:

- 2 ripe bananas peeled and sliced.
- 1/2 cup rolled oats.
- 1 cup low-fat yogurt
- 1/2 cup skim milk (or a dairy-free alternative)
- 1 tablespoon honey (optional for sweetness)
- 1/2 teaspoon vanilla extract
- 1/2 cup crushed ice
- 1 tablespoon ground flaxseed (optional for added nutrients)
- 1/2 cup fresh strawberries hulled and halved.

Cooking Instructions:

1. Place the sliced bananas, rolled oats, yogurt, skim milk (or alternative), honey (if using), and vanilla extract in a blender.

2. Add the crushed ice and blend until the mixture is smooth and creamy.

3. If desired, add ground flaxseed for an extra nutritional boost and blend again briefly to combine.

4. Pour the smoothie into two glasses and top with fresh strawberry halves.

5. Serve immediately and enjoy your calcium-fortified breakfast smoothie!

Nutritional Values:

- Calories: 230 kcal
- Protein: 8g
- Carbohydrates: 47g
- Dietary Fiber: 6g
- Sugars: 23g
- Fat: 2g

Cooking Tips: To make this smoothie even more calcium-rich, consider using yogurt fortified with extra calcium. Adjust the sweetness by adding more or less honey according to your taste preference. For variety, you can customize this smoothie with other fruits like blueberries, raspberries, or kiwi.

Recipe 2: Spinach and Feta Breakfast Quesadilla

Prep Time: 10 minutes - Cooking Time: 10 minutes - Number of Servings: 2

Ingredients:

- 2 large whole wheat tortillas
- 1 cup fresh spinach leaves
- 1/2 cup crumbled feta cheese
- 2 large eggs
- 1/4 cup skim milk (or a dairy-free alternative)
- Salt and pepper to taste
- Cooking spray or a touch of olive oil for the pan

Cooking Instructions:

1. In a mixing bowl, whisk the eggs, skim milk, salt, and pepper until well combined.

2. Heat a non-stick skillet over medium heat and lightly grease it with cooking spray or olive oil.

3. Pour half of the egg mixture into the skillet and cook until the edges start to set, about 2 minutes.

4. Place one tortilla on top of the eggs in the skillet.

5. Sprinkle half of the fresh spinach and half of the crumbled feta cheese on top of the tortilla.

6. Carefully flip the other half of the tortilla over to cover the spinach and cheese. Press down gently.

7. Cook for 2-3 minutes until the bottom is golden brown.

8. Flip the quesadilla and cook for 2-3 minutes until the other side is golden brown and the cheese is melted.

9. Remove from the skillet and repeat the process for the second quesadilla.

10. Slice each quesadilla into wedges and serve hot.

Nutritional Values:

- Calories: 340 kcal
- Protein: 18g
- Carbohydrates: 24g
- Dietary Fiber: 4g
- Sugars: 2g
- Fat: 20g

Cooking Tips: For a fluffier quesadilla filling, add a pinch of baking powder to the egg and milk mixture before whisking. The baking powder causes the egg mixture to rise slightly when cooked, creating a lighter texture that complements the crispiness of the tortilla.

Recipe 3: Berry-Almond Greek Yogurt Parfait

Prep Time: 5 minutes - Cooking Time: 0 minutes - Number of Servings: 2

Ingredients:

- 1 cup low-fat Greek yogurt
- 1/2 cup mixed berries (such as blueberries, strawberries, and raspberries)
- 1/4 cup sliced almonds.
- 2 tablespoons honey (optional for sweetness)
- 1/2 teaspoon vanilla extract

Cooking Instructions:

1. layering 1/4 cup of Greek yogurt at the bottom of two serving glasses or bowls.

2. Add a layer of mixed berries on top of the yogurt.

3. Sprinkle a portion of sliced almonds over the berries.

4. Drizzle honey (if using) over the almonds for a touch of sweetness.

5. Repeat the layering process with yogurt, berries, almonds, and honey.

6. Finish by adding a dash of vanilla extract to each parfait.

7. Serve immediately or refrigerate until ready to eat.

Nutritional Values:

- Calories: 280 kcal
- Protein: 15g
- Carbohydrates: 30g
- Dietary Fiber: 5g
- Sugars: 22g
- Fat: 12g
- Calcium: 300mg (30% DV)
- Vitamin C: 10mg (11% DV)

Cooking Tips: You can customize this parfait with your choice of berries and nuts for variety. Use unsweetened Greek yogurt if you prefer a lower-sugar option.

Recipe 4: Veggie and Cheese Omelet

Prep Time: 10 minutes - Cooking Time: 10 minutes - Number of Servings: 2

Ingredients:

- 4 large eggs
- 2 tablespoons low-fat milk (or a dairy-free alternative)
- Salt and pepper to taste
- 1/2 cup diced bell peppers (assorted colors)
- 1/2 cup diced tomatoes.
- 1/4 cup diced red onion.
- 1/4 cup shredded low-fat cheddar cheese.
- 1 tablespoon olive oil
- Fresh parsley for garnish (optional)

Cooking Instructions:

1. In a bowl, whisk together the eggs, low-fat milk, salt, and pepper until well beaten.

2. Heat olive oil in a non-stick skillet over medium heat.

3. Add diced bell peppers and red onion to the skillet. Sauté for 2-3 minutes until they begin to soften.

4. Add diced tomatoes to the skillet and continue to sauté for another 2 minutes until the vegetables are tender.

5. Pour the beaten egg mixture evenly over the sautéed vegetables.

6. Cook the omelet, gently lifting the edges with a spatula and tilting the skillet to allow uncooked eggs to flow underneath.

7. Once the omelet is mostly set but still slightly runny on top, sprinkle the shredded cheddar cheese over one-half of the omelet.

8. Carefully fold the other half of the omelet over the cheese side.

9. Cook for another 2 minutes until the cheese is melted and the omelet is cooked.

10. Slide the omelet onto a plate, garnish with fresh parsley if desired, and serve hot.

Nutritional Values:

- Calories: 280 kcal
- Protein: 16g
- Carbohydrates: 8g
- Dietary Fiber: 2g
- Sugars: 4g
- Fat: 21g

Cooking Tip: For an extra fluffy omelet, add a splash of carbonated water to the egg mixture before whisking, which introduces air bubbles and results in a lighter texture.

Recipe 5: Blueberry and Almond Chia Pudding

Prep Time: 5 minutes (plus chilling time) - **Cooking Time:** 0 minutes - **Number of Servings:** 2

Ingredients:

- 1/4 cup chia seeds
- 1 cup unsweetened almond milk (or any milk of your choice)
- 1/2 teaspoon vanilla extract
- 2 tablespoons honey (or maple syrup for a vegan option)
- 1/2 cup fresh blueberries
- 2 tablespoons sliced almonds.
- Fresh mint leaves for garnish (optional)

Cooking Instructions:

1. Combine chia seeds, unsweetened almond milk, vanilla extract, and honey in a mixing bowl. Stir well to combine.

2. Cover the bowl and refrigerate for at least 2 hours or overnight. This allows the chia seeds to absorb the liquid and form a pudding-like consistency.

3. Once the chia pudding is set, give it a good stir to make it creamy.

4. Divide the chia pudding between two serving glasses or bowls.

5. Top each serving with fresh blueberries and a sprinkle of sliced almonds.

6. Garnish with fresh mint leaves for flavor and color (optional).

7. Serve chilled and enjoy your nutritious and calcium-rich chia pudding!

Nutritional Values:

- Calories: 240 kcal
- Protein: 5g
- Carbohydrates: 34g
- Dietary Fiber: 9g
- Sugars: 19g
- Fat: 10g

Cooking Tips: Feel free to customize your chia pudding with other fruits like strawberries or raspberries. Adjust the sweetness by adding more or less honey or your preferred sweetener.

Recipe 6: Quinoa and Spinach Breakfast Bowl

Prep Time: 15 minutes - Cooking Time: 15 minutes - Number of Servings: 2

Ingredients:

- 1/2 cup quinoa rinsed and drained.
- 1 cup water or low-sodium vegetable broth
- 2 cups fresh spinach leaves
- 1/2 cup diced tomatoes.
- 1/4 cup crumbled feta cheese
- 2 large eggs
- 1 tablespoon olive oil
- Salt and pepper to taste
- Fresh basil leaves for garnish (optional)

Cooking Instructions:

1. Combine the quinoa and water (or vegetable broth) in a small saucepan. Bring to a boil, then reduce the heat to low, cover, and simmer for about 15 minutes until the quinoa is cooked and the liquid is absorbed. Fluff with a fork and set aside.

2. In a separate skillet, heat olive oil over medium heat. Add fresh spinach leaves and sauté until wilted, about 2-3 minutes. Season with salt and pepper to taste.

3. In the same skillet, push the wilted spinach to one side and crack the eggs into the other side. Cook until the egg whites are set, but the yolks are still slightly runny, about 3-4 minutes.

4. Divide the cooked quinoa between two serving bowls.

5. Top the quinoa with diced tomatoes, crumbled feta cheese, and sautéed spinach.

6. Carefully transfer a fried egg to each bowl.

7. Garnish with fresh basil leaves if desired.

8. Serve hot, mixing the runny egg yolk with the quinoa and creating a creamy, delicious sauce.

Nutritional Values:

- Calories: 340 kcal
- Protein: 14g
- Carbohydrates: 29g
- Dietary Fiber: 4g
- Sugars: 2g
- Fat: 19g

Cooking Tip: Toast the quinoa in the saucepan with a little olive oil for 2-3 minutes before adding water or broth; this enhances its nutty flavor and adds depth to the breakfast bowl.

Recipe 7: Whole-Grain Banana Pancakes

Prep Time: 10 minutes - Cooking Time: 15 minutes - Number of Servings: 2

Ingredients:

- 1 cup whole-grain flour
- 1 teaspoon baking powder
- 1/4 teaspoon baking soda
- 1/4 teaspoon salt
- 1 ripe banana, mashed.
- 1 large egg
- 1 cup low-fat buttermilk (or a dairy-free alternative)
- 1 tablespoon honey (optional for sweetness)
- 1/2 teaspoon vanilla extract
- Cooking spray or a touch of olive oil for the pan
- Fresh banana slices and a drizzle of honey for garnish (optional)

Cooking Instructions:

1. In a mixing bowl, whisk together whole-grain flour, baking powder, baking soda, and salt.

2. In a separate bowl, mash the ripe banana and add the egg, low-fat buttermilk, honey (if using), and vanilla extract. Mix until well combined.

3. Pour the wet ingredients into the dry ingredients and stir until combined. Do not overmix; a few lumps are okay.

4. Preheat a non-stick skillet over medium heat and lightly grease it with cooking spray or olive oil.

5. Pour 1/4 cup of the pancake batter onto the skillet for each pancake. Cook until bubbles form on the surface and the edges look set, about 2-3 minutes.

6. Flip the pancakes and cook for 1-2 minutes or until golden brown and cooked through.

7. Remove the pancakes from the skillet and keep them warm.

8. Serve the pancakes with fresh banana slices and a drizzle of honey if desired.

Nutritional Values:

- Calories: 320 kcal
- Protein: 10g
- Carbohydrates: 63g
- Dietary Fiber: 6g
- Sugars: 17g
- Fat: 4g

Cooking Tip: For extra fluffy pancakes, let the batter rest for 5-10 minutes after mixing; this allows the baking powder and soda to start working, creating air bubbles that result in lighter pancakes.

Recipe 8: Avocado and Tomato Toast with Poached Eggs

Prep Time: 10 minutes - Cooking Time: 10 minutes - Number of Servings: 2

Ingredients:

- 2 wholegrain bread slices (or your preferred type)
- 1 ripe avocado peeled and sliced.
- 1 large tomato, sliced.
- 2 large eggs
- 1 teaspoon white vinegar (for poaching eggs)
- Salt and pepper to taste
- Fresh cilantro or parsley for garnish (optional)

Cooking Instructions:

1. Toast the whole-grain bread slices until golden brown and crispy.

2. While the bread is toasting, prepare the poached eggs. Fill a large saucepan with about 2 inches of water and bring it to a gentle simmer. Add the white vinegar.

3. Crack one egg into a small bowl or ramekin. Create a gentle whirlpool in the simmering water by spooning it. Carefully slide the egg into the swirling water.

4. Poach the egg for 3-4 minutes for a runny yolk or longer for a firmer yolk. Use a slotted spoon to remove the poached egg and drain excess water. Repeat with the second egg.

5. Spread the sliced avocado evenly over the toasted bread slices.

6. Top the avocado with slices of fresh tomato.

7. Place one poached egg on each slice of toast.

8. Season with salt and pepper to taste and garnish with fresh cilantro or parsley if desired.

9. Serve immediately and enjoy this nutritious and calcium-rich breakfast!

Nutritional Values:

- Calories: 290 kcal
- Protein: 12g
- Carbohydrates: 22g
- Dietary Fiber: 9g
- Sugars: 2g
- Fat: 18g

Cooking Tip: Customize your toast with additional toppings like a sprinkle of feta cheese, red pepper flakes, or a drizzle of olive oil for extra flavor.

Recipe 9: Almond and Berry Breakfast Quinoa Bowl

Prep Time: 10 minutes - **Cooking Time:** 15 minutes - **Number of Servings:** 2

Ingredients:

- 1/2 cup quinoa rinsed and drained.
- 1 cup unsweetened almond milk (or any milk of your choice)
- 1/2 teaspoon vanilla extract
- 1/2 teaspoon ground cinnamon
- 1/4 cup sliced almonds.
- 1/2 cup mixed berries (such as blueberries, strawberries, and raspberries)
- 2 tablespoons honey (optional for sweetness)
- Fresh mint leaves for garnish (optional)

Cooking Instructions:

1. Combine the quinoa, almond milk, vanilla extract, and ground cinnamon in a saucepan. Bring to a boil.

2. Reduce the heat to low, cover, and simmer for about 15 minutes or until the quinoa is cooked and has absorbed the liquid. Fluff with a fork and set aside.

3. Toast the sliced almonds in a dry skillet over medium heat for 2-3 minutes until they are lightly browned and fragrant. Be careful not to burn them.

4. Divide the cooked quinoa between two serving bowls.

5. Top the quinoa with mixed berries and the toasted sliced almonds.

6. Drizzle honey (if using) over the top for a touch of sweetness.

7. Garnish with fresh mint leaves for added freshness and flavor (optional).

8. Serve warm and enjoy your calcium-rich breakfast quinoa bowl!

Nutritional Values:

- Calories: 320 kcal
- Protein: 8g
- Carbohydrates: 53g
- Dietary Fiber: 8g
- Sugars: 19g
- Fat: 10g

Cooking Tip: You can customize this breakfast bowl with other fruits or nuts.

Recipe 10: Cinnamon Apple Overnight Oats

Prep Time: 10 minutes (plus chilling time) - **Cooking Time:** 0 minutes - **Number of Servings:** 2

Ingredients:

- 1 cup rolled oats.
- 1 cup unsweetened almond milk (or any milk of your choice)
- 1/2 cup low-fat Greek yogurt
- 1 large apple grated or finely chopped.
- 1/2 teaspoon ground cinnamon
- 2 tablespoons honey (optional for sweetness)
- 1/4 cup chopped walnuts.
- Fresh apple slices for garnish (optional)

Cooking Instructions:

1. In a mixing bowl, combine rolled oats, unsweetened almond milk, low-fat Greek yogurt, grated or chopped apple, ground cinnamon, and honey (if using). Mix well to combine all ingredients.

2. Divide the oat mixture evenly between two mason jars or airtight containers.

3. Seal the jars or containers and refrigerate overnight, or for at least 4 hours, to allow the oats to soak and become creamy.

4. When ready to serve, give the overnight oats a good stir.

5. Top with chopped walnuts and garnish with fresh apple slices if desired.

6. Serve chilled, and enjoy your calcium-rich, non-cook breakfast!

Nutritional Values:

- Calories: 320 kcal
- Protein: 11g
- Carbohydrates: 54g
- Dietary Fiber: 7g
- Sugars: 22g
- Fat: 9g

Cooking Tip: Customize your overnight oats with toppings like berries, sliced bananas, or a sprinkle of ground flaxseed.

Chapter 4: Nourishing Soups and Salads - Savor the Flavors of Bone-Healthy Goodness

Welcome to Chapter 4 of the "Osteoporosis Diet Cookbook," where we'll explore the world of nourishing soups and salads that not only tantalize your taste buds but also contribute to your journey towards stronger bones. Soups and salads offer various flavors, textures, and vibrant, nutritious, and delicious ingredients.

In this chapter, we've compiled a collection of recipes that prioritize bone health while ensuring each bite is an experience. Soups and salads are packed with vitamins and minerals, making them an excellent opportunity to incorporate calcium ingredients, leafy greens, and lean proteins into your diet.

Whether indulging in a bowl of soup on an evening or enjoying a refreshing salad on a sunny day, our recipes provide diverse options for every occasion and palate. There's something for everyone, from hearty soups to salads bursting with colors and flavors.

So, get ready to savor the goodness of bone flavors as we dive into Chapter 4! Looking for a salad or a comforting bowl of soup? Look no further! This chapter is your go-to for inspiration. Treat your body to recipes that will keep your bones strong and resilient.

Let us embark on a journey through the world of nourishing soups and salads together, celebrating the pleasure of eating for bone health. Enjoy your meal!

Recipe 11: Creamy Broccoli and Cheddar Soup

Prep Time: 15 minutes - Cooking Time: 25 minutes - Number of Servings: 4

Ingredients:

- 2 tablespoons olive oil
- 1 small onion, chopped.
- 2 cloves garlic, minced.
- 4 cups fresh broccoli florets
- 4 cups low-sodium vegetable broth
- 1 cup low-fat milk (or a dairy-free alternative)
- 1 cup shredded low-fat cheddar cheese.
- Salt and pepper to taste
- Chopped fresh chives for garnish (optional)

Cooking Instructions:

1. Heat the olive oil over medium heat in a large pot. Add the chopped onion and sauté for 3-4 minutes until it becomes translucent.

2. Stir in the minced garlic and cook for 1-2 minutes until fragrant.

3. Add the fresh broccoli florets to the pot and sauté for another 2-3 minutes, stirring occasionally.

4. Pour the low-sodium vegetable broth, cover the pot, and simmer for about 15 minutes or until the broccoli is tender.

5. Using an immersion blender or a regular blender (in batches), carefully puree the soup until it's smooth.

6. Return the pureed soup to the pot and stir in the low-fat milk.

7. Heat the soup over low-medium heat, then gradually add the shredded low-fat cheddar cheese, stirring until it's fully melted, and the soup becomes creamy.

8. Season with salt and pepper to taste.

9. Serve hot, garnished with chopped fresh chives if desired.

Nutritional Values:

- Calories: 210 kcal
- Protein: 12g
- Carbohydrates: 15g
- Dietary Fiber: 4g
- Sugars: 7g
- Fat: 11g

Cooking Tips: Customize the soup by adding a pinch of nutmeg or a dash of cayenne pepper for extra flavor.

Recipe 12: Spinach and Strawberry Salad with Poppy Seed Dressing

Prep Time: 10 minutes - Cooking Time: 0 minutes - Number of Servings: 4

Ingredients:
For the Salad:

- 6 cups fresh baby spinach leaves
- 2 cups fresh strawberries hulled and sliced.
- 1/4 cup thinly sliced red onion.
- 1/4 cup chopped toasted almonds.
- 1/4 cup crumbled low-fat feta cheese.

For the Poppy Seed Dressing:

- 1/4 cup olive oil
- 2 tablespoons apple cider vinegar
- 1 tablespoon honey
- 1 teaspoon Dijon mustard
- 1 teaspoon poppy seeds
- Salt and pepper to taste

Salad Assembly Instructions:

1. combine the fresh baby spinach leaves, sliced strawberries, thinly sliced red onion, chopped toasted almonds, and crumbled low-fat feta cheese in a large salad bowl.

Poppy Seed Dressing Instructions:

1. In a separate small bowl, whisk together the olive oil, apple cider vinegar, honey, Dijon mustard, poppy seeds, salt, and pepper until well combined.

2. Taste the dressing and adjust the sweetness or tanginess by adding more honey or vinegar, if desired.

Salad Dressing Instructions:

1. Drizzle the poppy seed dressing over the spinach and strawberry salad before serving.

2. Gently toss the salad to evenly coat the ingredients with the dressing.

3. Serve immediately as a refreshing and calcium-rich salad.

Nutritional Values:

- Calories: 200 kcal
- Protein: 4g
- Carbohydrates: 17g
- Dietary Fiber: 4g
- Sugars: 10g
- Fat: 14g

Cooking Tips: To elevate the flavors and textures in your salad, chill the sliced strawberries and spinach leaves before assembling. This not only keeps the salad refreshing but also enhances the contrast between the crisp spinach, cool strawberries, and the tangy poppy seed dressing.

Recipe 13: Lentil and Kale Soup

Prep Time: 15 minutes - Cooking Time: 30 minutes - Number of Servings: 6

Ingredients:

- 1 cup dried green or brown lentils rinsed and drained.
- 8 cups low-sodium vegetable broth
- 2 tablespoons olive oil
- 1 onion, chopped.
- 3 cloves garlic, minced.
- 2 carrots, diced.
- 2 celery stalks, diced.
- 1 teaspoon ground cumin
- 1 teaspoon ground coriander
- 1/2 teaspoon smoked paprika.
- 1 bay leaf
- Salt and pepper to taste
- 4 cups fresh kale leaves, stems removed and chopped.
- Juice of 1 lemon
- Grated Parmesan cheese for garnish (optional)

Cooking Instructions:

1. Heat the olive oil over medium heat in a large pot. Add the chopped onion, minced garlic, carrots, and celery. Sauté for about 5 minutes or until the vegetables begin to soften.

2. Stir in the ground cumin, coriander, smoked paprika, and bay leaf. Cook for another minute until the spices become fragrant.

3. Add the rinsed and drained lentils to the pot. Pour in the low-sodium vegetable broth.

4. Bring the mixture to a boil, then reduce the heat to low, cover, and simmer for about 20-25 minutes or until the lentils are tender.

5. Season the soup with salt and pepper to taste.

6. Stir in the chopped kale and cook for 5 minutes or until the kale is wilted and tender.

7. Remove the bay leaf from the soup.

8. Just before serving, squeeze the juice of one lemon into the soup and stir well.

9. Serve hot, optionally garnished with grated Parmesan cheese for added flavor.

Nutritional Values:

- Calories: 220 kcal
- Protein: 11g
- Carbohydrates: 36g
- Dietary Fiber: 11g
- Sugars: 5g
- Fat: 5g

Recipe 14: Grilled Chicken and Quinoa Salad

Prep Time: 20 minutes - Cooking Time: 15 minutes - Number of Servings: 4

Ingredients:
For the Salad:

- 2 cups cooked quinoa (cooled)
- 2 cups grilled chicken breast, sliced.
- 2 cups mixed greens (such as spinach, arugula, and romaine)
- 1 cup cherry tomatoes, halved.
- 1/2 cup diced cucumber.
- 1/4 cup sliced red onion.
- 1/4 cup crumbled low-fat feta cheese.
- 1/4 cup sliced black olives (optional)

For the Balsamic Vinaigrette:

- 1/4 cup balsamic vinegar
- 1/4 cup olive oil
- 1 teaspoon Dijon mustard
- 1 clove garlic, minced.
- Salt and pepper to taste

Salad Assembly Instructions:

1. In a large salad bowl, combine the cooked and cooled quinoa, grilled chicken breast slices, mixed greens, cherry tomatoes, diced cucumber, sliced red onion, crumbled low-fat feta cheese, and sliced black olives (if using).

Balsamic Vinaigrette Instructions:

1. In a separate small bowl, whisk together the balsamic vinegar, olive oil, Dijon mustard, minced garlic, salt, and pepper until well combined.

2. Taste the dressing and adjust the seasoning if needed.

Salad Dressing Instructions:

1. Drizzle the balsamic vinaigrette over the salad just before serving.

2. Gently toss the salad to coat the ingredients with the dressing.

3. Serve immediately as a satisfying and calcium-rich salad.

Nutritional Values:

- Calories: 360 kcal
- Protein: 25g
- Carbohydrates: 21g
- Dietary Fiber: 3g
- Sugars: 4g
- Fat: 20g

Recipe 15: Butternut Squash and Kale Salad

Prep Time: 15 minutes - Cooking Time: 30 minutes - Number of Servings: 4

Ingredients:
For the Salad:

- 4 cups butternut squash peeled and diced.
- 2 tablespoons olive oil
- Salt and pepper to taste
- 8 cups fresh kale leaves, stems removed and chopped.
- 1/4 cup dried cranberries
- 1/4 cup chopped pecans.
- 1/4 cup crumbled low-fat goat cheese (optional)

For the Balsamic Maple Dressing:

- 3 tablespoons balsamic vinegar
- 2 tablespoons olive oil
- 1 tablespoon pure maple syrup
- 1 teaspoon Dijon mustard
- Salt and pepper to taste

Salad Assembly Instructions:

1. Preheat your oven to 400°F (200°C).

2. toss the diced butternut squash with olive oil, salt, and pepper in a large bowl.

3. Spread the butternut squash evenly on a baking sheet and roast for 25-30 minutes until tender and slightly caramelized. Stir once or twice during cooking.

4. While the butternut squash is roasting, prepare the kale. In a large salad bowl, combine the chopped kale, dried cranberries, chopped pecans, and crumbled low-fat goat cheese (if using).

Balsamic Maple Dressing Instructions:

1. In a separate small bowl, whisk together the balsamic vinegar, olive oil, pure maple syrup, Dijon mustard, salt, and pepper until well combined.

2. Taste the dressing and adjust the sweetness or tanginess by adding more maple syrup or vinegar, if desired.

Salad Dressing Instructions:

1. Drizzle the balsamic maple dressing over the kale salad before serving.

2. Gently toss the salad to coat the ingredients with the dressing.

3. Top the salad with the roasted butternut squash.

4. Serve immediately as a flavorful and calcium-rich salad.

Nutritional Values:

- Calories: 280 kcal
- Protein: 6g
- Carbohydrates: 38g
- Dietary Fiber: 6g

Recipe 16: Creamy Tomato Basil Soup

Prep Time: 15 minutes - Cooking Time: 25 minutes - Number of Servings: 4

Ingredients:

- 2 tablespoons olive oil
- 1 onion, chopped.
- 2 cloves garlic, minced.
- 2 cans (14 ounces each) diced tomatoes.
- 1 can (14 ounces) tomato sauce
- 2 cups low-sodium vegetable broth
- 1 teaspoon dried basil
- 1/2 teaspoon dried oregano
- Salt and pepper to taste
- 1/2 cup low-fat Greek yogurt (or plain yogurt)
- Fresh basil leaves for garnish (optional)

Cooking Instructions:

1. Heat the olive oil over medium heat in a large pot. Add the chopped onion and sauté for 3-4 minutes until it becomes translucent.

2. Stir in the minced garlic and cook for 1-2 minutes until fragrant.

3. Add the diced tomatoes (with their juices), tomato sauce, low-sodium vegetable broth, dried basil, dried oregano, salt, and pepper to the pot. Stir well to combine.

4. Bring the mixture to a boil, then reduce the heat to low, cover, and simmer for about 15-20 minutes, allowing the flavors to meld.

5. Using an immersion blender or a regular blender (in batches), carefully puree the soup until it's smooth.

6. Return the pureed soup to the pot and stir in the low-fat Greek yogurt until well combined.

7. Heat the soup over low-medium heat, stirring until heated.

8. Serve hot, garnished with fresh basil leaves if desired.

Nutritional Values:

- Calories: 170 kcal
- Protein: 6g
- Carbohydrates: 22g
- Dietary Fiber: 6g
- Sugars: 11g
- Fat: 7g

Cooking Tip: Customize your soup by adding a pinch of red pepper flakes for heat or a splash of cream for extra richness.

Recipe 17: Chickpea and Spinach Salad with Tahini Dressing

Prep Time: 15 minutes - Cooking Time: 0 minutes - Number of Servings: 4

Ingredients:
For the Salad:
- 2 cans (15 ounces each) chickpeas, drained and rinsed.
- 4 cups fresh baby spinach leaves
- 1 cup cherry tomatoes, halved.
- 1/2 cucumber, diced.
- 1/4 cup diced red onion.
- 1/4 cup chopped fresh parsley.
- 1/4 cup crumbled low-fat feta cheese (optional)

For the Tahini Dressing:
- 1/4 cup tahini (sesame paste)
- 2 tablespoons lemon juice
- 1 clove garlic, minced.
- 2 tablespoons water
- Salt and pepper to taste

Salad Assembly Instructions:
1. In a large salad bowl, combine the drained and rinsed chickpeas, fresh baby spinach leaves, halved cherry tomatoes, diced cucumber, diced red onion, chopped fresh parsley, and crumbled low-fat feta cheese (if using).

Tahini Dressing Instructions:
1. In a separate small bowl, whisk together the tahini, lemon juice, minced garlic, water, salt, and pepper until well combined.

2. Add more water to achieve your desired consistency if the dressing is too thick.

Salad Dressing Instructions:
1. Drizzle the tahini dressing over the salad just before serving.

2. Gently toss the salad to coat the ingredients with the dressing.

3. Serve immediately as a satisfying and calcium-rich salad.

Nutritional Values:
- Calories: 320 kcal
- Protein: 12g
- Carbohydrates: 40g
- Dietary Fiber: 11g
- Sugars: 9g
- Fat: 14g

Recipe 18: Quinoa and Black Bean Soup

Prep Time: 15 minutes - Cooking Time: 30 minutes - Number of Servings: 6

Ingredients:

- 1 cup quinoa rinsed and drained.
- 2 tablespoons olive oil
- 1 onion, chopped.
- 2 cloves garlic, minced.
- 1 red bell pepper, diced.
- 1 yellow bell pepper, diced.
- 1 can (15 ounces) black beans, drained and rinsed.
- 1 can (14 ounces) diced tomatoes.
- 6 cups low-sodium vegetable broth
- 1 teaspoon ground cumin
- 1 teaspoon chili powder
- Salt and pepper to taste
- Juice of 1 lime
- Chopped fresh cilantro for garnish (optional)
- Low-fat plain yogurt or sour cream for garnish (optional)

Cooking Instructions:

1. In a large pot, heat the olive oil over medium heat. Add the chopped onion and sauté for 3-4 minutes until it becomes translucent.

2. Stir in the minced garlic, red bell pepper, and yellow bell pepper. Cook for an additional 3-4 minutes until the peppers start to soften.

3. Add the rinsed and drained quinoa, black beans, diced tomatoes, low-sodium vegetable broth, ground cumin, chili powder, salt, and pepper to the pot. Stir well to combine.

4. Bring the mixture to a boil, then reduce the heat to low, cover, and simmer for about 20-25 minutes, or until the quinoa is cooked and the flavors meld.

5. Just before serving, squeeze the juice of one lime into the soup and stir well.

6. Serve hot, optionally garnished with chopped fresh cilantro and a dollop of low-fat plain yogurt or sour cream for added creaminess.

Nutritional Values:

- Calories: 290 kcal
- Protein: 9g
- Carbohydrates: 49g
- Dietary Fiber: 9g
- Sugars: 6g
- Fat: 7g

Recipe 19: Arugula and Roasted Beet Salad

Prep Time: 15 minutes - Cooking Time: 45 minutes (for roasting beets) - Number of Servings: 4

Ingredients:
For the Salad:

- 4 medium beets trimmed and scrubbed.
- 4 cups arugula leaves
- 1/2 cup crumbled low-fat goat cheese.
- 1/4 cup chopped walnuts, toasted.
- 1/4 cup thinly sliced red onion.

For the Balsamic Vinaigrette:

- 1/4 cup balsamic vinegar
- 1/4 cup olive oil
- 1 teaspoon Dijon mustard
- 1 clove garlic, minced.
- Salt and pepper to taste

Salad Assembly Instructions:

1. Preheat your oven to 400°F (200°C).

2. Wrap each beet individually in aluminum foil and place them on a baking sheet. Roast in the oven for about 45 minutes or until the beets are tender when pierced with a fork.

3. Allow the roasted beets to cool, then peel and cut them into thin slices or wedges.

4. Combine the arugula leaves, roasted beet slices, crumbled low-fat goat cheese, toasted chopped walnuts, and thinly sliced red onion in a large salad bowl.

Balsamic Vinaigrette Instructions:

1. In a separate small bowl, whisk together the balsamic vinegar, olive oil, Dijon mustard, minced garlic, salt, and pepper until well combined.

2. Taste the dressing and adjust the seasoning if needed.

Salad Dressing Instructions:

1. Drizzle the balsamic vinaigrette over the salad just before serving.

2. Gently toss the salad to coat the ingredients with the dressing.

3. Serve immediately as a flavorful and calcium-rich salad.

Nutritional Values:

- Calories: 220 kcal
- Protein: 7g
- Carbohydrates: 14g
- Dietary Fiber: 4g
- Sugars: 10g
- Fat: 16g

Recipe 20: Sweet Potato and Quinoa Salad

Prep Time: 15 minutes - Cooking Time: 20 minutes - Number of Servings: 4

Ingredients:
For the Salad:

- 2 cups cooked quinoa (cooled)
- 2 medium sweet potatoes peeled and diced.
- 2 tablespoons olive oil

For the Balsamic Maple Dressing:

- 1/4 cup balsamic vinegar
- 1/4 cup olive oil
- 2 tablespoons pure maple syrup
- 1 teaspoon Dijon mustard
- Salt and pepper to taste

Salad Assembly Instructions:

1. Preheat your oven to 400°F (200°C).

2. Toss the diced sweet potatoes with olive oil, salt, and pepper.

3. Spread the sweet potatoes in a single layer on a baking sheet and roast for about 20 minutes or until they are tender and slightly caramelized. Stir once while cooking.

4. In a large salad bowl, combine the cooked quinoa, roasted sweet potatoes, fresh baby spinach leaves, dried cranberries, toasted chopped pecans, and crumbled low-fat blue cheese (if using).

- Salt and pepper to taste
- 2 cups fresh baby spinach leaves
- 1/2 cup dried cranberries
- 1/4 cup chopped pecans, toasted.
- 1/4 cup crumbled low-fat blue cheese (optional)

Balsamic Maple Dressing Instructions:

1. In a separate small bowl, whisk together the balsamic vinegar, olive oil, pure maple syrup, Dijon mustard, salt, and pepper until well combined.

2. Taste the dressing and adjust the sweetness or tanginess by adding more maple syrup or vinegar, if desired.

Salad Dressing Instructions:

1. Drizzle the balsamic maple dressing over the salad just before serving.

2. Gently toss the salad to coat the ingredients with the dressing.

3. Serve immediately as a delicious calcium-rich salad.

Nutritional Values:

- Calories: 380 kcal
- Protein: 6g
- Carbohydrates: 51g
- Dietary Fiber: 7g
- Sugars: 17g
- Fat: 18g

Chapter 5: Wholesome Main Courses - Nourishing Your Bones with Every Bite

Welcome to Chapter 5 of the "Osteoporosis Diet Cookbook." This chapter will explore a collection of course recipes prioritizing bone health without compromising flavor. Main courses play a role in creating a meal, and we've carefully curated a range of nutritious and delicious options for you.

Within these pages, you'll find dishes that feature proteins, whole grains, and calcium-fortified ingredients – all for maintaining strong and healthy bones. Our main courses are designed to give your body nutrients and please your taste buds.

Whether you're cooking dinner for your loved ones or hosting a gathering, our recipes offer versatility and creativity. From succulent grilled proteins to grain-based dishes, there's something to suit everyone's preferences and dietary needs.

To help you master the art of preparing these dishes, we've included some cooking tips. These will ensure that each meal is both delightful and nutritious. You'll also find information to help you choose your main courses.

So get ready to nourish your bones with every bite as we embark on Chapter 5. These main courses are about filling your plate with the building blocks for strong and resilient bones while celebrating the joy of cooking well for better bone health. Let us begin an adventure exploring a variety of mouthwatering and healthy main dishes that can enhance your life one meal at a time.

Recipe 21: Baked Salmon with Lemon-Dill Sauce

Prep Time: 15 minutes - Cooking Time: 20 minutes - Number of Servings: 4

Ingredients:
For the Baked Salmon:

- 4 salmon fillets (about 6 ounces each)
- 2 tablespoons olive oil
- 1 teaspoon dried dill
- 1/2 teaspoon garlic powder
- Salt and pepper to taste
- Lemon wedges for garnish

For the Lemon-Dill Sauce:

- 1/2 cup low-fat Greek yogurt
- 2 tablespoons fresh lemon juice
- 1 teaspoon fresh dill, chopped.
- 1 teaspoon honey
- Salt and pepper to taste

Cooking Instructions:
Baked Salmon:

1. Preheat your oven to 375°F (190°C).

2. Place the salmon fillets on a baking sheet lined with parchment paper.

3. Mix the olive oil, dried dill, garlic powder, salt, and pepper in a small bowl.

4. Brush the mixture over the salmon fillets.

5. Bake in the oven for 15-20 minutes or until the salmon flakes easily with a fork.

Lemon-Dill Sauce:

1. While the salmon is baking, prepare the sauce. Combine the low-fat Greek yogurt, fresh lemon juice, fresh dill, honey, salt, and pepper in a small bowl. Mix until well combined.

Assembly:

1. Serve the baked salmon hot, garnished with lemon wedges, and drizzled with the lemon-dill sauce.

Nutritional Values:

- Calories: 320 kcal
- Protein: 35g
- Carbohydrates: 6g
- Dietary Fiber: 0.5g
- Sugars: 4g
- Fat: 18g

Cooking Tips: Pair this salmon dish with steamed broccoli or a side salad for a complete meal. Adjust the level of honey in the sauce to balance the sweetness according to your preference. Salmon is a great source of calcium, vitamin D, and omega-3 fatty acids, all important for bone health.

Recipe 22: Quinoa-Stuffed Bell Peppers

Prep Time: 20 minutes - Cooking Time: 45 minutes - Number of Servings: 4

Ingredients:

For the Stuffed Bell Peppers:

- 4 large bell peppers, any color
- 1 cup quinoa rinsed and drained.
- 2 cups low-sodium vegetable broth
- 1 can (15 ounces) black beans, drained and rinsed.
- 1 cup corn kernels (fresh, frozen, or canned)
- 1 cup diced tomatoes.
- 1 teaspoon chili powder
- 1/2 teaspoon ground cumin
- Salt and pepper to taste
- 1/2 cup shredded low-fat cheddar cheese (optional)

For the Avocado-Cilantro Sauce:

- 1 ripe avocado
- 1/4 cup fresh cilantro leaves
- Juice of 1 lime
- 1 clove garlic, minced.
- Salt and pepper to taste
- Water (to reach desired consistency)

Cooking Instructions:

Stuffed Bell Peppers:

1. Preheat your oven to 375°F (190°C).

2. Cut the tops off the bell peppers and remove the seeds and membranes. Rinse them under cold water and set aside.

3. combine the quinoa and low-sodium vegetable broth in a medium saucepan. Bring to a boil, then reduce the heat to low, cover, and simmer for 15-20 minutes or until the quinoa is cooked and the liquid is absorbed.

4. combine the cooked quinoa, black beans, corn kernels, diced tomatoes, chili powder, ground cumin, salt, and pepper in a large mixing bowl. Mix well.

5. Stuff the bell peppers with the quinoa mixture and place them in a baking dish.

6. If desired, sprinkle the shredded low-fat cheddar cheese on top of each stuffed bell pepper.

7. Cover the baking dish with aluminum foil and bake in the oven for 25-30 minutes or until the bell peppers are tender.

Avocado-Cilantro Sauce:

1. While the stuffed bell peppers are baking, prepare the sauce. Combine the ripe avocado, fresh cilantro leaves, lime juice, minced garlic, salt, and pepper in a blender or food processor.

2. Add water as needed to reach your desired sauce consistency. Blend until smooth.

Assembly:

1. Serve hot stuffed bell peppers drizzled with the avocado-cilantro sauce.

Nutritional Values:

- Calories: 380 kcal
- Protein: 15g
- Carbohydrates: 65g
- Dietary Fiber: 13g
- Sugars: 6g

Recipe 23: Spinach and Mushroom Stuffed Chicken Breast

Prep Time: 20 minutes - Cooking Time: 25 minutes - Number of Servings: 4

Ingredients:

For the Stuffed Chicken:

- 4 boneless, skinless chicken breasts
- Salt and pepper to taste
- 2 cups fresh spinach leaves
- 1 cup sliced mushrooms.
- 1/2 cup low-fat feta cheese
- 1 tablespoon olive oil
- 1 teaspoon dried oregano
- 1 teaspoon garlic powder
- Toothpicks for security.

For the Balsamic Glaze:

- 1/4 cup balsamic vinegar
- 1 tablespoon honey
- Salt and pepper to taste

Cooking Instructions:

Stuffed Chicken:

1. Preheat your oven to 375°F (190°C).

2. Season each chicken breast with salt and pepper.

3. Heat olive oil in a skillet over medium-high heat. Add sliced mushrooms and sauté for about 5 minutes until they release moisture and become tender. Set them aside.

4. In the same skillet, add fresh spinach leaves and sauté for about 2-3 minutes until they wilt. Remove from heat.

5. Combine sautéed mushrooms, wilted spinach, crumbled low-fat feta cheese, dried oregano, and garlic powder in a mixing bowl.

6. Slice a pocket into each chicken breast without cutting through the other side.

7. Stuff each chicken breast with the spinach-mushroom mixture, using toothpicks to secure the openings.

8. Place the stuffed chicken breasts in a baking dish.

Balsamic Glaze:

1. In a small saucepan, combine balsamic vinegar and honey. Bring to a simmer over medium heat, then reduce the heat and cook for about 5 minutes until the glaze thickens slightly. Season with salt and pepper.

Assembly:

1. Drizzle the balsamic glaze over the stuffed chicken breasts.

2. Bake in the oven for about 20-25 minutes or until the chicken is cooked and no longer pink in the center.

Nutritional Values:

- Calories: 250 kcal
- Protein: 32g
- Carbohydrates: 10g
- Dietary Fiber: 2g
- Sugars: 6g

Recipe 24: Lentil and Vegetable Stir-Fry

Prep Time: 15 minutes - Cooking Time: 20 minutes - Number of Servings: 4

Ingredients:

For the Stir-Fry:

- 1 cup dry green or brown lentils rinsed and drained.
- 2 cups water
- 2 tablespoons olive oil
- 1 onion, chopped.
- 2 cloves garlic, minced.
- 2 cups mixed vegetables (bell peppers, broccoli, snap peas, carrots, etc.), sliced.
- 1 cup snow peas, trimmed.
- 1/4 cup low-sodium soy sauce
- 2 tablespoons rice vinegar
- 1 tablespoon honey
- 1 teaspoon grated fresh ginger.
- Salt and pepper to taste
- Sesame seeds for garnish (optional)

Cooking Instructions:

Stir-Fry:

1. In a medium saucepan, combine the rinsed lentils and water. Bring to a boil, then reduce the heat to low, cover, and simmer for 15-20 minutes or until the lentils are tender but not mushy. Drain any excess water and set aside.

2. Heat the olive oil over medium-high heat in a large skillet or wok. Add the chopped onion and sauté for 2-3 minutes until it becomes translucent.

3. Add the minced garlic, mixed vegetables, and snow peas to the skillet. Stir-fry for about 5-7 minutes or until the vegetables are crisp-tender.

4. Stir in the cooked lentils and mix well with the vegetables.

Sauce:

1. Whisk the low-sodium soy sauce, rice vinegar, honey, grated fresh ginger, salt, and pepper in a small bowl.

Assembly:

1. Pour the sauce into the skillet over the lentil and vegetable mixture.

2. Stir-fry for 2-3 minutes, allowing the flavors to meld and the sauce to coat the ingredients.

3. Serve hot, garnished with sesame seeds if desired.

Nutritional Values:

- Calories: 320 kcal
- Protein: 16g
- Carbohydrates: 52g
- Dietary Fiber: 14g
- Sugars: 9g
- Fat: 7g

Recipe 25: Grilled Chicken and Vegetable Skewers with Yogurt-Herb Sauce

Prep Time: 20 minutes - Cooking Time: 15 minutes - Number of Servings: 4

Ingredients:

For the Skewers:

- 1-pound boneless, skinless chicken breasts cut into chunks
- 2 bell peppers (assorted colors), cut into chunks.
- 1 red onion, cut into chunks.
- 1 zucchini, sliced into rounds.
- 8 cherry tomatoes
- Wooden skewers, soaked in water for 30 minutes (to prevent burning)

For the Yogurt-Herb Sauce:

- 1 cup low-fat Greek yogurt
- 2 tablespoons fresh lemon juice
- 1/4 cup fresh herbs (such as parsley, cilantro, and mint), chopped.
- 2 cloves garlic, minced.
- Salt and pepper to taste

Cooking Instructions:

Skewers:

1. Preheat your grill to medium-high heat.

2. Thread the chicken chunks, bell pepper chunks, red onion chunks, zucchini rounds, and cherry tomatoes onto the soaked wooden skewers in an alternating pattern.

3. Brush the skewers with olive oil and season with salt and pepper.

4. Grill the skewers for 10-15 minutes, turning occasionally, or until the chicken is cooked and the vegetables are tender and lightly charred.

Yogurt-Herb Sauce:

1. While the skewers are grilling, prepare the sauce. Combine the low-fat Greek yogurt, fresh lemon juice, chopped fresh herbs, minced garlic, salt, and pepper in a bowl. Mix well.

Assembly:

1. Serve the grilled chicken and vegetable skewers hot, accompanied by the yogurt-herb sauce for dipping.

Nutritional Values:

- Calories: 270 kcal
- Protein: 32g
- Carbohydrates: 18g
- Dietary Fiber: 4g
- Sugars: 10g
- Fat: 7g

Cooking Tips: Customize your skewers with your favorite vegetables and herbs.

Recipe 26: Eggplant Parmesan

Prep Time: 30 minutes - Cooking Time: 40 minutes - Number of Servings: 4

Ingredients:

For the Eggplant:

- 2 medium eggplants, thinly sliced into rounds.
- 2 cups whole wheat breadcrumbs
- 1 cup grated Parmesan cheese.
- 2 eggs, beaten.
- Salt and pepper to taste
- Cooking spray

For the Tomato Sauce:

- 2 cans (14 ounces each) crushed tomatoes.
- 2 cloves garlic, minced.
- 1 teaspoon dried basil
- 1 teaspoon dried oregano
- Salt and pepper to taste

For Assembling:

- 2 cups shredded part-skim mozzarella cheese.
- Fresh basil leaves for garnish (optional)

Cooking Instructions:

Eggplant:

1. Preheat your oven to 375°F (190°C).

2. In a shallow bowl, combine the whole wheat breadcrumbs, grated Parmesan cheese, salt, and pepper.

3. Dip each eggplant slice into the beaten eggs and the breadcrumb mixture, ensuring it's evenly coated.

4. Place the breaded eggplant slices on a baking sheet sprayed with cooking spray.

5. Bake in the oven for 15-20 minutes or until the eggplant is tender and the coating is golden brown.

Tomato Sauce:

1. In a saucepan, Combine the crushed tomatoes, minced garlic, dried basil, dried oregano, salt, and pepper. Bring to a simmer over medium heat and cook for about 10 minutes, stirring occasionally.

Assembly:

1. In a baking dish, spread a small amount of tomato sauce to coat the bottom.

2. Place a layer of baked eggplant slices on the sauce.

3. Add a layer of shredded part-skim mozzarella cheese.

4. Repeat the layers until all the eggplant slices are used, finishing with a layer of mozzarella cheese.

5. Bake in the oven for about 20-25 minutes or until the cheese is melted and bubbly.

Nutritional Values:

- Calories: 380 kcal
- Protein: 20g
- Carbohydrates: 35g
- Dietary Fiber: 11g
- Sugars: 12g
- Fat: 18g

Recipe 27: Tofu and Broccoli Stir-Fry

Prep Time: 20 minutes - Cooking Time: 15 minutes - Number of Servings: 4

Ingredients:
For the Stir-Fry:
- 14 ounces extra-firm tofu pressed and cubed.
- 2 tablespoons low-sodium soy sauce
- 1 tablespoon sesame oil
- 1 tablespoon cornstarch
- 2 tablespoons canola oil
- 2 cups broccoli florets
- 1 red bell pepper, sliced.
- 1 yellow bell pepper, sliced.
- 1 carrot thinly sliced.
- 2 cloves garlic, minced.
- 1 teaspoon grated fresh ginger.
- Salt and pepper to taste

For the Sauce:
- 1/4 cup low-sodium soy sauce
- 2 tablespoons honey
- 1 tablespoon rice vinegar
- 1 teaspoon cornstarch

Cooking Instructions:
Stir-Fry:

1. In a bowl, combine the cubed tofu, 2 tablespoons of low-sodium soy sauce, sesame oil, and 1 tablespoon of cornstarch. Toss to coat the tofu evenly.

2. Heat canola oil in a large skillet or wok over medium-high heat. Add the tofu and cook for about 5-7 minutes, turning occasionally, until it's crispy and golden brown. Remove tofu from the skillet and set aside.

3. Add the minced garlic and grated ginger in the same skillet. Sauté for about 1 minute until fragrant.

4. Add the broccoli florets, red bell pepper slices, yellow bell pepper slices, and carrot slices to the skillet. Stir-fry for about 5 minutes until the vegetables are tender-crisp.

Sauce:

1. In a small bowl, whisk together 1/4 cup of low-sodium soy sauce, honey, rice vinegar, and 1 teaspoon of cornstarch until well combined.

Assembly:

1. Return the cooked tofu to the skillet with the vegetables.

2. Pour the sauce over the tofu and vegetables. Stir-fry for 2-3 minutes, thickening the sauce and coating the ingredients.

3. Season with salt and pepper to taste.

4. Serve hot over brown rice or whole wheat noodles if desired.

Nutritional Values:
- Calories: 280 kcal
- Protein: 12g
- Carbohydrates: 22g
- Dietary Fiber: 5g
- Sugars: 12g
- Fat: 17g

Recipe 28: Beef and Vegetable Stir-Fry

Prep Time: 20 minutes - Cooking Time: 15 minutes - Number of Servings: 4

Ingredients:

For the Stir-Fry:

- 1-pound lean beef (such as sirloin or flank steak), thinly sliced
- 2 tablespoons low-sodium soy sauce
- 1 tablespoon cornstarch
- 2 tablespoons canola oil
- 2 cups broccoli florets
- 1 red bell pepper, sliced.
- 1 yellow bell pepper, sliced.
- 1 carrot thinly sliced.
- 2 cloves garlic, minced.
- 1 teaspoon grated fresh ginger.
- Salt and pepper to taste

For the Sauce:

- 1/4 cup low-sodium soy sauce
- 2 tablespoons honey
- 1 tablespoon rice vinegar
- 1 teaspoon cornstarch

Cooking Instructions:

Stir-Fry:

1. In a bowl, combine the thinly sliced beef, 2 tablespoons of low-sodium soy sauce, and 1 tablespoon of cornstarch. Toss to coat the beef evenly.

2. Heat canola oil in a large skillet or wok over medium-high heat. Add the beef and cook for about 2-3 minutes, stirring occasionally, until it's browned. Remove beef from the skillet and set aside.

3. In the same skillet, add minced garlic and grated ginger. Sauté for about 1 minute until fragrant.

4. Add the broccoli florets, red bell pepper slices, yellow bell pepper slices, and carrot slices to the skillet. Stir-fry for about 5 minutes until the vegetables are tender-crisp.

Sauce:

1. In a small bowl, whisk together 1/4 cup of low-sodium soy sauce, honey, rice vinegar, and 1 teaspoon of cornstarch until well combined.

Assembly:

1. Return the cooked beef to the skillet with the vegetables.

2. Pour the sauce over the beef and vegetables. Stir-fry for 2-3 minutes, thickening the sauce and coating the ingredients.

3. Season with salt and pepper to taste.

4. Serve hot over brown rice or whole wheat noodles if desired.

Nutritional Values:

- Calories: 290 kcal
- Protein: 24g
- Carbohydrates: 21g
- Dietary Fiber: 4g
- Sugars: 11g

Recipe 29: Chickpea and Spinach Curry

Prep Time: 15 minutes - Cooking Time: 25 minutes - Number of Servings: 4

Ingredients:
For the Chickpea and Spinach Curry:

- 2 tablespoons olive oil
- 1 onion finely chopped.
- 2 cloves garlic, minced.
- 1inch piece of fresh ginger, minced.
- 2 teaspoons curry powder
- 1 teaspoon ground cumin
- 1 teaspoon ground coriander
- 1/2 teaspoon ground turmeric
- 1/2 teaspoon paprika
- 1 can (15 ounces) chickpeas, drained and rinsed.
- 1 can (14 ounces) diced tomatoes.
- 1 cup vegetable broth
- 2 cups fresh baby spinach leaves
- Salt and pepper to taste
- Fresh cilantro leaves for garnish (optional)

For Serving:

- Cooked brown rice or whole wheat couscous.

Cooking Instructions:

Chickpea and Spinach Curry:

1. Heat the olive oil over medium heat in a large skillet or saucepan. Add the chopped onion and sauté for about 3-4 minutes until it becomes translucent.

2. Add the minced garlic and ginger, and sauté for another minute until fragrant.

3. Stir in the curry powder, ground cumin, coriander, turmeric, and paprika. Cook for about 1 minute to toast the spices.

4. Add the chickpeas, diced tomatoes, and vegetable broth to the skillet. Stir well to combine.

5. Simmer the curry mixture for about 10-15 minutes, allowing the flavors to meld and the sauce to thicken.

6. Add the fresh baby spinach leaves to the skillet and cook for 2-3 minutes until the spinach wilts.

Assembly:

1. Season the chickpea and spinach curry with salt and pepper to taste.

2. Serve the curry with hot, overcooked brown rice or whole wheat couscous.

3. Garnish with fresh cilantro leaves if desired.

Nutritional Values:

- Calories: 220 kcal
- Protein: 8g
- Carbohydrates: 32g
- Dietary Fiber: 8g
- Sugars: 6g
- Fat: 7g

Recipe 30: Quinoa and Black Bean Stuffed Bell Peppers

Prep Time: 20 minutes - Cooking Time: 45 minutes - Number of Servings: 4

Ingredients:

For the Stuffed Bell Peppers:

- 4 large bell peppers, any color
- 1 cup quinoa rinsed and drained.
- 2 cups low-sodium vegetable broth
- 1 can (15 ounces) black beans, drained and rinsed.
- 1 cup corn kernels (fresh, frozen, or canned)
- 1 cup diced tomatoes.
- 1 teaspoon chili powder
- 1/2 teaspoon ground cumin
- Salt and pepper to taste
- 1/2 cup shredded low-fat cheddar cheese (optional)

For the Avocado-Cilantro Sauce:

- 1 ripe avocado
- 1/4 cup fresh cilantro leaves
- Juice of 1 lime
- 1 clove garlic, minced.
- Salt and pepper to taste
- Water (to reach desired consistency)

Cooking Instructions:

Stuffed Bell Peppers:

1. Preheat your oven to 375°F (190°C).

2. Cut the tops off the bell peppers and remove the seeds and membranes. Rinse them under cold water and set aside.

3. Combine the quinoa and low-sodium vegetable broth in a medium saucepan. Bring to a boil, then reduce the heat to low, cover, and simmer for 15-20 minutes, or until the quinoa is cooked and the liquid is absorbed.

4. Combine the cooked quinoa, black beans, corn kernels, diced tomatoes, chili powder, ground cumin, salt, and pepper in a large mixing bowl. Mix well.

5. Stuff the bell peppers with the quinoa mixture.

6. If desired, sprinkle the shredded low-fat cheddar cheese on top of each stuffed bell pepper.

7. Cover the baking dish with aluminum foil and bake in the oven for 25-30 minutes or until the bell peppers are tender.

Avocado-Cilantro Sauce:

1. While the stuffed bell peppers are baking, prepare the sauce. Combine the ripe avocado, fresh cilantro leaves, lime juice, minced garlic, salt, and pepper in a blender or food processor.

2. Add water as needed to reach your desired sauce consistency. Blend until smooth.

Nutritional Values:

- Calories: 380 kcal
- Protein: 15g
- Carbohydrates: 65g
- Dietary Fiber: 13g
- Sugars: 6g
- Fat: 9g

Chapter 6: Sides and Snacks for Strong Bones - Bite-Sized Delights That Bolster Your Bone Health

Here, we'll discover a selection of side dishes and snacks that satisfy your taste buds and contribute to the strength and maintenance of your bones. Sides and snacks play a role in ensuring you receive rounded and satisfying nutrition daily.

In this chapter, we have curated a collection of recipes showcasing vegetables, fruits, nuts, and seeds – known for their bone-strengthening properties. These dishes are crafted to be both delicious and nutritious, offering an array of textures and flavors that will please your palate.

Preparing our recipes is designed to maximize flavor and nutritional value. We have included cooking tips so you can make the most of these recipes, whether cooking for yourself or sharing them with loved ones. Additionally, nutritional information is provided to help you choose your sides and snacks.

So, let us embark on this journey of bite delights that promote bone health together! Whether you serve these dishes as side dishes to your courses or enjoy them as nutritious snacks, this chapter will help you discover tasty and nourishing options that promote strong and resilient bones.

Come join us in celebrating the pleasures of eating for improved bone health and relish the opportunities that await you in Chapter 6.

Enjoy your meal!

Recipe 31: Mango Salsa

Prep Time: 15 minutes - Number of Servings: 4

Ingredients:

- 2 ripe mangos, diced.
- 1/2 red onion finely chopped.
- 1 red bell pepper, diced.
- 1/4 cup fresh cilantro, chopped.
- Juice of 2 limes
- Salt and pepper to taste
- 1 jalapeño pepper, seeded and finely chopped (optional for heat)

Cooking Instructions:

1. Combine diced mangos, finely chopped red onion, bell pepper, and fresh cilantro.

2. Squeeze the juice of 2 limes over the mixture.

3. If you prefer a bit of heat, add the finely chopped jalapeño pepper.

4. Season with salt and pepper and toss to combine.

Nutritional Values:

- Calories: 70 kcal
- Protein: 1g
- Carbohydrates: 18g
- Dietary Fiber: 2g
- Sugars: 14g
- Fat: 0.5g

Cooking Tips: Serve this refreshing salsa with grilled chicken or fish for a tropical twist. Adjust the heat by including or omitting the jalapeño pepper to suit your preference.

Recipe 32: Avocado and Tomato Bruschetta

Prep Time: 15 minutes - Cooking Time: 5 minutes - Number of Servings: 4

Ingredients:

- 2 ripe avocados, diced.
- 2 tomatoes, diced.
- 2 cloves garlic, minced.
- 1/4 cup fresh basil leaves, chopped.
- 2 tablespoons extra-virgin olive oil
- 1 tablespoon balsamic vinegar
- Salt and pepper to taste
- 1 French baguette, sliced.

Cooking Instructions:

1. Combine diced avocados, tomatoes, minced garlic, and chopped fresh basil in a bowl.

2. Drizzle extra-virgin olive oil and balsamic vinegar over the mixture.

3. Season with salt and pepper, and gently toss to combine.

4. Toast the slices of French baguette in the oven or on a grill until they're lightly golden and crisp.

5. Serve the avocado and tomato mixture on the toasted baguette slices.

Nutritional Values:

- Calories: 230 kcal
- Protein: 4g
- Carbohydrates: 23g
- Dietary Fiber: 5g
- Sugars: 2g
- Fat: 15g

Cooking Tips: For added flavor, rub the toasted baguette slices with a garlic clove before topping with the avocado and tomato mixture. You can also drizzle some honey over the bruschetta for sweetness.

Recipe 33: Spinach and Artichoke Dip

Prep Time: 10 minutes - Cooking Time: 20 minutes - Number of Servings: 6

Ingredients:

- 1 (10ounce) package of frozen chopped spinach, thawed and drained
- 1 (14ounce) can artichoke hearts, drained and chopped
- 1 cup low-fat Greek yogurt
- 1 cup low-fat cream cheese
- 1/2 cup grated Parmesan cheese.
- 1/2 cup shredded low-fat mozzarella cheese.
- 2 cloves garlic, minced.
- Salt and pepper to taste
- Whole wheat pita bread or tortilla chips for dipping

Cooking Instructions:

1. Preheat your oven to 375°F (190°C).

2. In a mixing bowl, combine the drained, chopped spinach, chopped artichoke hearts, low-fat Greek yogurt, low-fat cream cheese, grated Parmesan cheese, shredded low-fat mozzarella cheese, minced garlic, salt, and pepper. Mix until well combined.

3. Transfer the mixture to a baking dish.

4. Bake in the oven for about 20 minutes or until the dip is hot and bubbly and the top is lightly golden.

5. For dipping, Serve the spinach and artichoke dip with whole wheat pita bread or tortilla chips.

Nutritional Values:

- Calories: 140 kcal
- Protein: 11g
- Carbohydrates: 7g
- Dietary Fiber: 2g
- Sugars: 2g
- Fat: 8g

Cooking Tips: Squeeze the excess moisture from the thawed spinach to prevent the dip from becoming too watery. You can also sprinkle a little extra grated Parmesan cheese on top of the dip before baking for a nice cheesy crust.

Recipe 34: Walnut and Cranberry Quinoa Salad

Prep Time: 15 minutes - Cooking Time: 20 minutes - Number of Servings: 4

Ingredients:

- 1 cup quinoa rinsed and drained.
- 2 cups water
- 1/2 cup dried cranberries
- 1/2 cup chopped walnuts.
- 1/4 cup fresh parsley, chopped.
- 2 tablespoons olive oil
- 2 tablespoons fresh lemon juice
- Salt and pepper to taste
- 1/2 teaspoon ground cumin (optional)

Cooking Instructions:

1. In a medium saucepan, combine the quinoa and water. Bring to a boil, then reduce the heat to low, cover, and simmer for 15-20 minutes, or until the quinoa is cooked and the water is absorbed. Fluff with a fork and let it cool.

2. combine the cooked quinoa, dried cranberries, chopped walnuts, and chopped fresh parsley in a large bowl.

3. Drizzle with olive oil and fresh lemon juice.

4. Season with salt and pepper. For added flavor, sprinkle ground cumin over the salad.

5. Toss to combine all the ingredients. Serve chilled.

Nutritional Values:

- Calories: 340 kcal
- Protein: 7g
- Carbohydrates: 47g
- Dietary Fiber: 5g
- Sugars: 9g
- Fat: 15g

Cooking Tips: Customize the salad by adding your favorite herbs, such as mint or basil, for extra freshness. You can substitute other dried fruits like raisins or apricots if you prefer different flavors in your salad.

Recipe 35: Guacamole with Veggie Sticks

Prep Time: 15 minutes - Number of Servings: 4

Ingredients:

- 3 ripe avocados peeled and pitted.
- 1 tomato, diced.
- 1/4 cup red onion finely chopped.
- 1/4 cup fresh cilantro, chopped.
- Juice of 1 lime
- Salt and pepper to taste
- Assorted veggie sticks for dipping (carrots, celery, cucumber)

Assembly Instructions:

1. Mash the peeled and pitted avocados with a fork until you reach your desired guacamole consistency (smooth or chunky).

2. Stir in the diced tomato, finely chopped red onion, fresh cilantro, and lime juice.

3. Season with salt and pepper and mix until all ingredients are well combined.

4. Serve the guacamole with assorted veggie sticks for dipping.

Nutritional Values:

- Calories: 180 kcal
- Protein: 3g
- Carbohydrates: 15g
- Dietary Fiber: 10g
- Sugars: 2g
- Fat: 14g

Cooking Tips: To prevent guacamole from turning brown, press plastic wrap directly onto the surface of the dip to reduce exposure to air. Experiment with additional ingredients like diced jalapeño for some heat or diced mango for sweetness.

Recipe 36: Baked Sweet Potato Chips

Prep Time: 10 minutes - Cooking Time: 20 minutes - Number of Servings: 4

Ingredients:

- 2 large, sweet potatoes peeled and thinly sliced.
- 2 tablespoons olive oil
- 1 teaspoon paprika
- 1/2 teaspoon garlic powder
- Salt and pepper to taste

Cooking Instructions:

1. Preheat your oven to 425°F (220°C).

2. In a large bowl, toss the sweet potato slices with olive oil, paprika, garlic powder, salt, and pepper until they are evenly coated.

3. Arrange the seasoned sweet potato slices on a baking sheet in a single layer.

4. Bake in the preheated oven for approximately 15-20 minutes or until the chips are crispy and slightly golden, flipping them halfway through the cooking time.

5. Remove them from the oven and let them cool slightly before serving.

Nutritional Values:

- Calories: 160 kcal
- Protein: 2g
- Carbohydrates: 22g
- Dietary Fiber: 4g
- Sugars: 6g
- Fat: 7g

Cooking Tips: Make sure to slice the sweet potatoes thinly and uniformly for even cooking. Keep an eye on them as they bake; they can go from golden to burnt quickly.

Recipe 37: Mixed Berry Smoothie Bowl

Prep Time: 10 minutes - Number of Servings: 2

Ingredients:

- 2 cups mixed berries (strawberries, blueberries, raspberries)
- 1 ripe banana
- 1/2 cup low-fat Greek yogurt
- 1/4 cup almond milk (or any preferred milk)
- 2 tablespoons honey (optional)
- Toppings: sliced bananas, chia seeds, granola, shredded coconut, or additional berries

Assembly Instructions:

1. In a blender, combine the mixed berries, ripe banana, low-fat Greek yogurt, almond milk, and honey (if desired).

2. Blend until the mixture is smooth and creamy. If it's too thick, you can add more almond milk.

3. Pour the smoothie into two bowls.

4. Add your favorite toppings, such as sliced bananas, chia seeds, granola, shredded coconut, or additional berries.

Nutritional Values:

- Calories: 160 kcal
- Protein: 6g
- Carbohydrates: 36g
- Dietary Fiber: 5g
- Sugars: 24g
- Fat: 1g

Cooking Tips: Customize your smoothie bowl with your favorite toppings for added texture and flavor. You can freeze some of the berries ahead of time to make the smoothie even more refreshing and thick.

Recipe 38: Quinoa Salad with Cranberries and Almonds

Prep Time: 15 minutes - Number of Servings: 4

Ingredients:

- 1 cup quinoa rinsed and drained.
- 2 cups water
- 1/2 cup dried cranberries
- 1/2 cup sliced almonds.
- 1/4 cup fresh parsley, chopped.
- 2 tablespoons olive oil
- 2 tablespoons fresh lemon juice
- Salt and pepper to taste

Assembly Instructions:

1. In a medium saucepan, combine the quinoa and water. Bring to a boil, then reduce the heat to low, cover, and simmer for about 15 minutes until the quinoa is cooked and the water is absorbed. Fluff with a fork and let it cool.

2. combine the cooked quinoa, dried cranberries, sliced almonds, and chopped fresh parsley in a large bowl.

3. Drizzle with olive oil and fresh lemon juice.

4. Season with salt and pepper and toss to combine all the ingredients.

Nutritional Values:

- Calories: 280 kcal
- Protein: 7g
- Carbohydrates: 38g
- Dietary Fiber: 5g
- Sugars: 9g
- Fat: 11g

Cooking Tips: Add diced cucumber or cherry tomatoes for extra freshness and crunch. Add grilled chicken or chickpeas for protein to complete the meal.

Recipe 39: Carrot and Raisin Salad

Prep Time: 10 minutes - Number of Servings: 4

Ingredients:

- 4 cups shredded carrots.
- 1/2 cup raisins
- 1/4 cup plain Greek yogurt.
- 2 tablespoons honey
- 1 tablespoon lemon juice
- 1/4 teaspoon ground cinnamon
- 1/4 teaspoon ground nutmeg

Assembly Instructions:

1. In a large bowl, combine the shredded carrots and raisins.

2. Whisk together the plain Greek yogurt, honey, lemon juice, ground cinnamon, and ground nutmeg in a separate bowl.

3. Pour the yogurt mixture over the carrots and raisins.

4. Toss to coat evenly.

5. Chill the salad in the refrigerator for 30 minutes before serving.

Nutritional Values:

- Calories: 140 kcal
- Protein: 3g
- Carbohydrates: 33g
- Dietary Fiber: 4g
- Sugars: 24g
- Fat: 0.5g

Cooking Tips: Adjust the sweetness by adding more or less honey according to your taste preference. Add a handful of chopped nuts like almonds or pecans for extra crunch and healthy fats.

Recipe 40: Almond and Date Energy Bites

Prep Time: 15 minutes - Chilling Time: 30 minutes - Number of Servings: 12

Ingredients:

- 1 cup rolled oats.
- 1/2 cup almond butter
- 1/3 cup honey
- 1/2 cup chopped dates.
- 1/2 cup chopped almonds.
- 1/4 cup ground flaxseed
- 1 teaspoon vanilla extract
- Pinch of salt
- Optional: shredded coconut for rolling

Assembly Instructions:

1. In a large bowl, combine rolled oats, almond butter, honey, chopped dates, chopped almonds, ground flaxseed, vanilla extract, and a pinch of salt. Mix well.

2. Form the mixture into bite-sized balls using your hands.

3. Optional: Roll the energy bites in shredded coconut for added flavor.

4. Place the energy bites on a baking sheet lined with parchment paper and refrigerate for 30 minutes to firm up.

Nutritional Values:

- Calories: 150 kcal
- Protein: 4g
- Carbohydrates: 18g
- Dietary Fiber: 3g
- Sugars: 10g
- Fat: 8g

Cooking Tips: Customize these energy bites by adding dark chocolate chips, dried cranberries, or your favorite nuts. Store them in an airtight container in the refrigerator for longer freshness.

Chapter 7: Desserts and Treats - Satisfy Your Sweet Tooth with Bone-Healthy Delights

Welcome to Chapter 7 of the "Osteoporosis Diet Cookbook," where we'll explore the realm of desserts and treats specially designed for individuals with osteoporosis. We believe indulging in satisfying desserts can be a part of a bone diet without sacrificing flavor or nutrition.

In this chapter, we've curated a collection of dessert recipes that are not rich in calcium but have reduced sugar content. These desserts are guilt-free and delectable, allowing you to enjoy your treats while promoting good bone health.

We understand the significance of desserts and treats in our lives. Recognize that a balanced diet should include moments of indulgence. From luscious and creamy delights to creative fruit-based confections, our recipes exemplify that desserts can be nourishing and delightful.

Our recipes are thoughtfully crafted with your well-being and satisfaction in mind. We've included cooking tips to help you master the art of creating bone desserts that you and your loved ones can relish. Additionally, nutritional information is provided to assist you in making choices about your creations.

So, let us delve into Chapter 7 and embark on a journey through the world of desserts and treats that will appease your cravings while supporting your quest for resilient bones.

Indulge yourself with a variety of desserts and treats that are not only delicious but also promote bone health. This chapter will guide you to guilt indulgence, from creamy parfaits to tantalizing fruity delights.

Join us in celebrating the pleasure of savoring these bone delights, proving that taking care of your bones can also be an experience for your taste buds.

Recipe 41: Creamy Berry Parfait

Prep Time: 15 minutes - Cooking Time: None - Number of Servings: 4

Ingredients:

- 2 cups low-fat Greek yogurt
- 1 cup mixed berries (strawberries, blueberries, raspberries)
- 2 tablespoons honey
- 1/4 cup granola

Assembly Instructions:

1. Layer low-fat Greek yogurt, mixed berries, and a drizzle of honey in a bowl.
2. Repeat the layers as desired.
3. Top with granola for added texture and crunch.

Nutritional Values:

- Calories: 180 kcal
- Protein: 12g
- Carbohydrates: 30g
- Dietary Fiber: 3g
- Sugars: 19g
- Fat: 2g

Cooking Tips: This versatile dessert uses fresh or frozen mixed berries, depending on the season. Feel free to add a sprinkle of chopped nuts for extra flavor and healthy fats.

Recipe 42: Chia Seed Pudding with Almonds and Dates

Prep Time: 5 minutes - Chilling Time: 2-4 hours - Number of Servings: 4

Ingredients:

- 1/2 cup chia seeds
- 2 cups almond milk (or any preferred milk)
- 1/4 cup chopped almonds.
- 1/4 cup chopped dates.
- 2 tablespoons honey (optional)
- 1 teaspoon vanilla extract
- Pinch of salt

Assembly Instructions:

1. In a bowl, combine chia seeds and almond milk. Stir well.

2. Add chopped almonds, dates, honey (if desired), vanilla extract, and a pinch of salt. Mix thoroughly.

3. Cover the bowl and refrigerate for at least 2-4 hours, or until the chia seeds absorb the liquid and the mixture thickens.

4. Before serving, stir the pudding to distribute the ingredients evenly.

Nutritional Values:

- Calories: 220 kcal
- Protein: 6g
- Carbohydrates: 27g
- Dietary Fiber: 10g
- Sugars: 13g
- Fat: 11g

Cooking Tips: Customize your chia pudding with your favorite toppings like fresh berries, sliced bananas, or a sprinkle of cinnamon. Adjust the sweetness by adding more or less honey to suit your taste.

Recipe 43: Frozen Banana Bites

Prep Time: 10 minutes - Freezing Time: 2 hours - Number of Servings: 4

Ingredients:

- 2 ripe bananas
- 1/4 cup low-fat Greek yogurt
- 2 tablespoons almond butter (or any nut butter)
- 1/4 cup dark chocolate chips
- 1/4 cup chopped nuts (e.g., almonds, walnuts)
- 1/4 teaspoon vanilla extract

Assembly Instructions:

1. Slice the ripe bananas into rounds.

2. Mix low-fat Greek yogurt, almond butter, dark chocolate chips, chopped nuts, and vanilla extract until well combined.

3. Lay out half of the banana rounds on a baking sheet lined with parchment paper.

4. Spoon a small amount of the yogurt mixture onto each banana round.

5. Top with the remaining banana rounds to create bite-sized sandwiches.

6. Freeze for at least 2 hours until they are firm.

Nutritional Values:

- Calories: 220 kcal
- Protein: 5g
- Carbohydrates: 26g
- Dietary Fiber: 4g
- Sugars: 14g
- Fat: 12g

Cooking Tips: Customize your frozen banana bites by rolling them in shredded coconut or crushed nuts before freezing for added texture. Feel free to use white or milk chocolate chips if you prefer a sweeter treat.

Recipe 44: Chocolate Avocado Mousse

Prep Time: 10 minutes - Chilling Time: 2 hours - Number of Servings: 4

Ingredients:

- 2 ripe avocados peeled and pitted.
- 1/4 cup unsweetened cocoa powder
- 1/4 cup honey or maple syrup
- 1 teaspoon vanilla extract
- Pinch of salt
- Fresh berries for garnish (optional)

Assembly Instructions:

1. In a food processor, combine the peeled and pitted avocados, unsweetened cocoa powder, honey or maple syrup, vanilla extract, and a pinch of salt.

2. Blend until the mixture is smooth and creamy.

3. Divide the chocolate avocado mousse into serving dishes or glasses.

4. Refrigerate for at least 2 hours to chill and set.

5. Before serving, garnish with fresh berries if desired.

Nutritional Values:

- Calories: 220 kcal
- Protein: 3g
- Carbohydrates: 28g
- Dietary Fiber: 7g
- Sugars: 18g
- Fat: 13g

Cooking Tips: Make sure your avocados are ripe for a smoother texture. Adjust the sweetness by adding more or less honey or maple syrup to taste.

Recipe 45: Almond and Oat Cookies

Prep Time: 15 minutes - Cooking Time: 12 minutes - Number of Servings: 12 cookies!

Ingredients:

- 1 cup rolled oats.
- 1/2 cup almond butter
- 1/4 cup honey or maple syrup
- 1/4 cup chopped almonds.
- 1/4 cup dried cranberries
- 1/4 teaspoon baking soda
- 1/4 teaspoon vanilla extract
- Pinch of salt

Cooking Instructions:

1. Preheat your oven to 350°F (175°C) and line a baking sheet with parchment paper.

2. Combine rolled oats, almond butter, honey, or maple syrup, chopped almonds, dried cranberries, baking soda, vanilla extract, and a pinch of salt. Mix until well combined.

3. Scoop tablespoon-sized portions of the dough onto the prepared baking sheet, spacing them apart.

4. Use a fork to flatten each cookie slightly, creating a crisscross pattern.

5. Bake in the oven for about 12 minutes or until the cookies are lightly golden.

6. Allow the cookies to cool on the baking sheet for a few minutes before transferring them to a wire rack to cool completely.

Nutritional Values:

- Calories: 130 kcal
- Protein: 3g
- Carbohydrates: 14g
- Dietary Fiber: 2g
- Sugars: 8g
- Fat: 7g

Cooking Tips: Customize your cookies by adding dark chocolate chips, chopped dried apricots, or your favorite nuts. Be careful not to overbake; the cookies will continue to firm up as they cool.

Recipe 46: Greek Yogurt and Honey Popsicles

Prep Time: 10 minutes - Freezing Time: 4-6 hours - Number of Servings: 6 popsicles!

Ingredients:

- 2 cups low-fat Greek yogurt
- 1/4 cup honey
- 1 teaspoon vanilla extract
- 1 cup mixed berries (strawberries, blueberries, raspberries)

Assembly Instructions:

1. Mix low-fat Greek yogurt, honey, and vanilla extract until well combined.

2. Mix the yogurt into popsicle molds, filling each mold halfway.

3. Add mixed berries to each mold, pushing them into the yogurt mixture.

4. Top each mold with more yogurt mixture, leaving a small gap at the top.

5. Insert popsicle sticks into each mold.

6. Freeze for 4-6 hours or until the popsicles are firm.

Nutritional Values:

- Calories: 120 kcal
- Protein: 7g
- Carbohydrates: 20g
- Dietary Fiber: 1g
- Sugars: 17g
- Fat: 1g

Cooking Tips: You can use any combination of fresh or frozen berries for variety. To easily remove the popsicles from the molds, run them under warm water for a few seconds.

Recipe 47: Mango and Coconut Chia Popsicles

Prep Time: 10 minutes - Freezing Time: 4-6 hours - Number of Servings: 6 popsicles!

Ingredients:

- 1 cup diced mango (fresh or frozen)
- 1/2 cup coconut milk
- 2 tablespoons chia seeds
- 2 tablespoons honey or maple syrup
- 1/2 teaspoon vanilla extract
- Pinch of salt

Assembly Instructions:

1. Combine diced mango, coconut milk, chia seeds, honey or maple syrup, vanilla extract, and a pinch of salt in a blender.

2. Blend until you have a smooth mixture.

3. Pour the mango-coconut mixture into popsicle molds, filling each mold almost to the top.

4. Insert popsicle sticks into each mold.

5. Freeze for 4-6 hours or until the popsicles are solid.

Nutritional Values:

- Calories: 90 kcal
- Protein: 1g
- Carbohydrates: 16g
- Dietary Fiber: 2g
- Sugars: 12g
- Fat: 3g

Cooking Tips: Feel free to squeeze lime juice for a zesty twist. If using fresh mango, ensure its ripe for the best flavor and sweetness.

Recipe 48: Berry and Yogurt Bark

Prep Time: 10 minutes - Freezing Time: 3-4 hours - Number of Servings: 6

Ingredients:

- 2 cups low-fat Greek yogurt
- 1/4 cup honey
- 1 teaspoon vanilla extract
- 1 cup mixed berries (strawberries, blueberries, raspberries)
- 2 tablespoons chopped almonds.
- 2 tablespoons shredded coconut

Assembly Instructions:

1. Mix low-fat Greek yogurt, honey, and vanilla extract until well combined.

2. Line a baking sheet with parchment paper.

3. Pour the yogurt mixture onto the parchment paper, spreading it evenly to form a rectangle.

4. Sprinkle mixed berries, chopped almonds, and shredded coconut evenly over the yogurt.

5. Gently press the toppings into the yogurt.

6. Freeze for 3-4 hours or until the bark is completely frozen.

7. Break the bark into pieces and serve.

Nutritional Values:

- Calories: 120 kcal
- Protein: 6g
- Carbohydrates: 20g
- Dietary Fiber: 2g
- Sugars: 17g
- Fat: 2g

Cooking Tips: For variety, experiment with different toppings like sliced kiwi, pomegranate seeds, or crushed nuts. Store any leftover bark in an airtight container in the freezer.

Recipe 49: Frozen Yogurt Banana Pops

Prep Time: 10 minutes - Freezing Time: 2 hours - Number of Servings: 4

Ingredients:

- 2 ripe bananas, peeled and cut in half.
- 1/2 cup low-fat Greek yogurt
- 1/4 cup unsweetened shredded coconut
- 1/4 cup chopped pistachios.
- 2 tablespoons honey
- 1/4 teaspoon vanilla extract
- Wooden popsicle sticks

Assembly Instructions:

1. Insert wooden popsicle sticks into the cut end of each banana half.

2. Mix low-fat Greek yogurt, honey, vanilla extract, and a pinch of salt in a shallow dish.

3. Dip each banana pop into the yogurt mixture, ensuring an even coating.

4. Roll the coated banana pops in unsweetened shredded coconut and chopped pistachios.

5. Place the coated banana pops on a baking sheet lined with parchment paper.

6. Freeze for at least 2 hours or until the pops are firm.

Nutritional Values:

- Calories: 160 kcal
- Protein: 4g
- Carbohydrates: 28g
- Dietary Fiber: 3g
- Sugars: 16g
- Fat: 6g

Cooking Tips: Customize your banana pops using toppings like crushed graham crackers or mini chocolate chips. To simplify dipping, you can slice the banana halves in half lengthwise before inserting the popsicle sticks.

Recipe 50: Cinnamon Apple Crisp

Prep Time: 15 minutes - Baking Time: 40 minutes - Number of Servings: 6

Ingredients:

Filling:

- 4 cups sliced apples (such as Granny Smith or Honeycrisp)
- 1 tablespoon lemon juice
- 2 tablespoons honey or maple syrup
- 1/2 teaspoon ground cinnamon
- 1/4 teaspoon ground nutmeg

Topping:

- 1 cup rolled oats.
- 1/2 cup whole wheat flour
- 1/4 cup chopped walnuts.
- 2 tablespoons honey
- 2 tablespoons melted coconut oil.
- 1/2 teaspoon ground cinnamon
- Pinch of salt

Baking Instructions:

1. Preheat your oven to 350°F (175°C).

2. In a large bowl, combine sliced apples, lemon juice, honey or maple syrup, ground cinnamon, and ground nutmeg. Toss until the apples are evenly coated.

3. Transfer the apple mixture to a greased baking dish.

4. In a separate bowl, combine rolled oats, whole wheat flour, chopped walnuts, honey, melted coconut oil, ground cinnamon, and a pinch of salt. Mix until it forms a crumbly topping.

5. Sprinkle the oat topping evenly over the apples in the baking dish.

6. Bake in the preheated oven for about 35-40 minutes or until the topping is golden brown and the apples are tender.

7. Allow the apple crisp to cool slightly before serving.

Nutritional Values:

- Calories: 260 kcal
- Protein: 4g
- Carbohydrates: 45g
- Dietary Fiber: 6g
- Sugars: 24g
- Fat: 10g

Chapter 8: Meal Plans and Tips for Success - Navigating Your Bone-Healthy Journey

Welcome to Chapter 8 of "The Osteoporosis Diet Cookbook." Here, we offer guidance on creating meal plans and incorporating recipes that promote bones into your everyday life. This chapter focuses on practicality, providing sample meal plans and many tips and strategies to make your journey toward bone health seamless and enjoyable.

We understand the importance of planning and consistent effort to maintain a diet supporting bones. We have developed sample meal plans tailored to preferences and lifestyles. Whether you follow a vegetarian diet or enjoy meat-based dishes. Have dietary restrictions; these meal plans are designed to offer well-rounded nutrition while prioritizing the health of your bones.

In addition to the meal plans, this chapter is packed with tips and strategies that will help you effortlessly incorporate bone recipes into your daily routine. We will share insights on grocery shopping, efficient meal prepping, and making choices when dining out. We aim to equip you with knowledge and tools to make consuming bone-healthy meals natural.

By the end of this chapter, you will have a roadmap for nourishing your body with nutrients daily. We aim to ensure that attaining resilient bones is attainable but also sustainable and enjoyable.

So, let us embark on this journey together and confidently navigate the path towards improving bone health. Whether you follow our suggested meal plans or incorporate tips and strategies, rest assured that each step brings you closer to a happier version of yourself. Come join us in celebrating the art of meal planning and embracing the simplicity of incorporating bone choices into your life. Here's to your success in your endeavor for bone health!

Sample Meal Plan 1: Balanced Diet

Day 1:

- Breakfast: Greek yogurt parfait with mixed berries and a sprinkle of granola.

- Lunch: Spinach and feta stuffed chicken breast with a side salad.

- Dinner: Baked salmon with quinoa and steamed broccoli.

- Snack: Sliced cucumber and carrot sticks with hummus.

Day 2:

- Breakfast: Oatmeal topped with sliced bananas and almonds.

- Lunch: Lentil and vegetable soup with a whole-grain roll.

- Dinner: Grilled tofu stir-fry with brown rice and snap peas.

- Snack: Low-fat cottage cheese with pineapple chunks.

Day 3:

- Breakfast: Scrambled eggs with spinach and tomatoes.

- Lunch: Quinoa salad with chickpeas, cucumbers, and a lemon-tahini dressing.

- Dinner: Baked cod with sweet potato and roasted asparagus.

- Snack: Apple slices with almond butter.

Sample Meal Plan 2: Vegetarian and Calcium-Rich

Day 1:

- Breakfast: Greek yogurt and mixed berry smoothie.

- Lunch: Spinach and feta stuffed bell peppers.

- Dinner: Lentil curry with brown rice.

- Snack: Sliced pear with a handful of almonds.

Day 2:

- Breakfast: Spinach and mushroom omelet with a side of whole-grain toast.

- Lunch: Quinoa and black bean salad with avocado.

- Dinner: Baked tofu with broccoli and quinoa.

- Snack: Carrot and celery sticks with hummus.

Day 3:

- Breakfast: Cottage cheese with sliced peaches and a drizzle of honey.

- Lunch: Greek salad with chickpeas and a lemon-tahini dressing.

- Dinner: Vegetable stir-fry with tofu and brown rice.

- Snack: Low-fat yogurt with mixed nuts.

Sample Meal Plan 3: Vegan and Calcium-Focused

Day 1:

- Breakfast: Chia pudding made with almond milk and topped with berries.

- Lunch: Vegan lentil soup with a side of whole-grain crackers.

- Dinner: Roasted vegetable and quinoa bowl with tahini dressing.

- Snack: Sliced cucumber with balsamic vinegar.

Day 2:

- Breakfast: Vegan smoothie bowl with spinach, banana, and almond butter.

- Lunch: Chickpea salad with mixed greens and lemon-tahini dressing.

- Dinner: Stir-fried tempeh with broccoli and brown rice.

- Snack: Almond and date energy bites.

Day 3:

- Breakfast: Vegan tofu scrambled with spinach and tomatoes.

- Lunch: Vegan quinoa and black bean bowl with avocado.

- Dinner: Vegan vegetable curry with quinoa.

- Snack: Sliced apple with almond butter.

Sample Meal Plan 4: Mediterranean Diet for Bone Health

Day 1:

- Breakfast: Greek yogurt with honey and walnuts.

- Lunch: Mediterranean quinoa salad with tomatoes, cucumbers, olives, and feta cheese.

- Dinner: Grilled chicken breast with roasted vegetables and quinoa.

- Snack: Hummus with whole-grain pita and carrot sticks.

Day 2:

- Breakfast: Whole-grain toast with avocado and poached eggs.

- Lunch: Lentil and vegetable soup with a side of mixed greens.

- Dinner: Baked salmon with a lemon-dill sauce, served with brown rice and steamed broccoli.

- Snack: Greek yogurt with fresh berries.

Day 3:

- Breakfast: Spinach and feta omelet with a whole-grain English muffin.

- Lunch: Falafel and tabbouleh salad with tahini dressing.

- Dinner: Mediterranean-style grilled tofu with quinoa and grilled asparagus.

- Snack: Sliced cucumber and cherry tomatoes with tzatziki.

Sample Meal Plan 5: Plant-Based and Calcium-Rich

Day 1:

- Breakfast: Smoothie with almond milk, kale, banana, and chia seeds.

- Lunch: Vegan lentil and vegetable stew with whole-grain bread.

- Dinner: Vegan stir-fried tempeh with broccoli and brown rice.

- Snack: Sliced pear with almond butter.

Day 2:

- Breakfast: Vegan chia pudding made with coconut milk and topped with mixed berries.

- Lunch: Vegan chickpea and spinach curry with quinoa.

- Dinner: Vegan roasted vegetable and tofu bowl with tahini dressing.

- Snack: Vegan almond and date energy bites.

Day 3:

- Breakfast: Vegan avocado toast with tomato and nutritional yeast.

- Lunch: Vegan Mediterranean quinoa salad with chickpeas, olives, and tahini dressing.

- Dinner: Vegan vegetable stir-fry with tofu and brown rice.

- Snack: Vegan mixed nuts and dried fruit.

Sample Meal Plan 6: Low-Carb and Bone-Healthy

Day 1:

- Breakfast: Scrambled eggs with spinach and mushrooms.

- Lunch: Grilled chicken breast with mixed greens and avocado.

- Dinner: Baked salmon with garlic butter, served with roasted asparagus.

- Snack: Celery sticks with almond butter.

Day 2:

- Breakfast: Greek yogurt with sliced strawberries and a drizzle of honey.

- Lunch: Turkey and vegetable stir-fry with a side of cauliflower rice.

- Dinner: Grilled shrimp with a spinach and walnut salad.

- Snack: Sliced cucumber with hummus.

Day 3:

- Breakfast: Omelet with tomatoes, bell peppers, and feta cheese.

- Lunch: Tuna salad with mixed greens and a vinaigrette dressing.

- Dinner: Beef and broccoli stir-fry with a side of steamed broccoli.

- Snack: Cottage cheese with pineapple chunks.

Get your FREE Meal Planner here:

https://prosebooks.com/meal-planner

Chapter 9: Bonus Recipes – Culinary Delights for Extraordinary Bone Health

Welcome to Chapter 9 of your "Osteoporosis Diet Cookbook." Here, we invite you to discover a collection of recipes that promote bone health. These bonus recipes are like the icing on the cake for your bone journey, offering a delightful range of options for breakfast, lunch, main courses, snacks, and desserts.

Within this chapter, we have curated bonus recipes to cater to tastes and occasions. These recipes provide opportunities to nourish your body with nutrient-rich ingredients while savoring the pleasures of good food. These recipes, from breakfasts to satisfying courses, are designed to please your palate and enhance your journey toward better bone health.

Our bonus recipes come complete with instructions, cooking tips, and nutritional information. This ensures that every dish you prepare becomes a masterpiece in terms of both flavor and nutrition. Whether you're seeking a start to the day, a tasty lunch option, a main course, or a treat to satisfy your sweet cravings. Rest assured that there's something here that will excite your taste buds.

Come join us in savoring the flavors and nutritional advantages these bonus recipes bring to your dining table. Here's to your success and culinary exploration as you strive for more resilient bones.

Enjoy your meal!

Recipe 51: Greek Yogurt Pancakes

Prep Time: 10 minutes – Cooking Time: 10 minutes – Number of Servings: 4

Ingredients:

- 1 cup Greek yogurt
- 2 large eggs
- ½ cup whole wheat flour
- 1 teaspoon baking powder
- ½ teaspoon vanilla extract
- 1 tablespoon honey
- Pinch of salt
- Fresh berries for garnish (optional)

Cooking Instructions:

1. Whisk together Greek yogurt, eggs, whole wheat flour, baking powder, vanilla extract, honey, and a pinch of salt until you have a smooth batter.

2. Heat a non-stick skillet or griddle over medium heat and lightly grease it with cooking spray or oil.

3. Pour ¼ cup portions of the batter onto the hot skillet to form pancakes. Cook until bubbles form on the surface (about 2-3 minutes).

4. Flip the pancakes and cook for another 2-3 minutes or until golden brown.

5. Serve the pancakes warmly, garnished with fresh berries if desired.

Nutritional Values:

- Calories: 180 kcal
- Protein: 12g
- Carbohydrates: 20g
- Dietary Fiber: 3g
- Sugars: 6g
- Fat: 6g

Cooking Tips: Let the batter rest for a few minutes before cooking fluffier pancakes. Add a touch of cinnamon or lemon zest for extra flavor.

Recipe 52: Quinoa Salad with Roasted Vegetables

Prep Time: 15 minutes – Cooking Time: 25 minutes – Number of Servings: 4

Ingredients:
For the Salad:

- 1 cup quinoa rinsed and drained.
- 2 cups mixed vegetables (bell peppers, zucchini, cherry tomatoes)
- 2 tablespoons olive oil
- 1 teaspoon dried thyme
- Salt and pepper to taste
- 1/4 cup crumbled feta cheese (optional)

For the Dressing:

- 3 tablespoons olive oil
- 2 tablespoons lemon juice
- 1 teaspoon honey or maple syrup
- 1 clove garlic, minced.
- Salt and pepper to taste

Cooking Instructions:

1. Preheat your oven to 400°F (200°C).

2. In a bowl, toss the mixed vegetables with 2 tablespoons of olive oil, dried thyme, salt, and pepper.

3. Spread the vegetables on a baking sheet and roast in the oven for about 20-25 minutes or until they are tender and slightly caramelized. Stir them occasionally for even cooking.

4. While roasting the vegetables, cook the quinoa according to the instructions. Once cooked, fluff it with a fork and let it cool.

5. In a small bowl, whisk together the ingredients for the dressing: 3 tablespoons of olive oil, lemon juice, honey or maple syrup, minced garlic, salt, and pepper.

6. Combine the cooked quinoa and roasted vegetables in a large salad bowl. Pour the dressing over the salad and toss to coat evenly.

7. If desired, sprinkle crumbled feta cheese over the top.

8. Serve the salad warm or at room temperature.

Nutritional Values:

- Calories: 320 kcal
- Protein: 6g
- Carbohydrates: 38g
- Dietary Fiber: 5g
- Sugars: 4g
- Fat: 16g

Recipe 53: Lemon Herb Grilled Chicken

Prep Time: 15 minutes - Marinating Time: 30 minutes - Cooking Time: 15 minutes - Number of Servings: 4

Ingredients:

- 4 boneless, skinless chicken breasts
- Zest and juice of 1 lemon.
- 2 cloves garlic, minced.
- 2 tablespoons fresh parsley, chopped.
- 1 tablespoon fresh thyme leaves
- 1 tablespoon olive oil
- Salt and pepper to taste

Cooking Instructions:

1. In a bowl, combine the lemon zest, lemon juice, minced garlic, chopped parsley, fresh thyme leaves, olive oil, salt, and pepper to make the marinade.

2. Place the chicken breasts in a resealable plastic bag or a shallow dish. Pour the marinade over the chicken, ensuring it's well coated. Seal the bag or cover the dish and refrigerate for at least 30 minutes (or longer for more flavor).

3. Preheat your grill to medium-high heat.

4. Remove the chicken from the marinade and let any excess drip off.

5. Grill the chicken for 6-7 minutes per side or until it's cooked through and has grill marks.

6. Remove the chicken from the grill and let it rest for a few minutes before serving.

7. Garnish with additional fresh herbs and lemon slices if desired.

Nutritional Values:

- Calories: 190 kcal
- Protein: 28g
- Carbohydrates: 2g
- Dietary Fiber: 0g
- Sugars: 0g
- Fat: 7g

Cooking Tips: Use a meat thermometer to ensure the chicken reaches an internal temperature of 165°F (74°C). Grilled vegetables or a simple salad make great side dishes for this flavorful chicken.

Recipe 54: Roasted Chickpeas Snack

Prep Time: 5 minutes - Cooking Time: 25 minutes - Number of Servings: 4

Ingredients:

- 2 (15ounce) cans of chickpeas, drained and rinsed
- 2 tablespoons olive oil
- 1 teaspoon paprika
- 1/2 teaspoon ground cumin
- 1/2 teaspoon garlic powder
- 1/2 teaspoon salt
- 1/4 teaspoon black pepper
- 1/4 teaspoon cayenne pepper (adjust to taste)

Cooking Instructions:

1. Preheat your oven to 400°F (200°C).

2. Rinse and drain the chickpeas, spread them on a clean kitchen towel, and pat them dry. Remove any loose skin.

3. In a large bowl, Toss the chickpeas with olive oil, paprika, ground cumin, garlic powder, salt, black pepper, and cayenne pepper.

4. Spread the seasoned chickpeas on a baking sheet in a single layer.

5. Roast in the preheated oven for 20-25 minutes or until the chickpeas are crispy, shaking the pan every 10 minutes for even cooking.

6. Remove the roasted chickpeas from the oven and let them cool before serving.

Nutritional Values:

- Calories: 230 kcal
- Protein: 8g
- Carbohydrates: 31g
- Dietary Fiber: 8g
- Sugars: 0g
- Fat: 9g

Cooking Tips: Customize the seasoning to your taste. You can try spices like curry powder, smoked paprika, or rosemary. Store any leftover roasted chickpeas in an airtight container for a crunchy snack.

Recipe 55: Berry and Almond Parfait

Prep Time: 10 minutes - Number of Servings: 2

Ingredients:

- 1 cup Greek yogurt
- 1 cup mixed berries (strawberries, blueberries, raspberries)
- 2 tablespoons honey
- 2 tablespoons sliced almonds.
- 1/2 teaspoon vanilla extract

Assembly Instructions:

1. Mix Greek yogurt with honey and vanilla extract until well combined in a bowl.

2. Layer the yogurt mixture, mixed berries, and sliced almonds in serving glasses or bowls.

3. Repeat the layers until the glasses are filled, finishing with a sprinkle of sliced almonds.

4. Serve immediately as a delightful and healthy dessert or snack.

Nutritional Values:

- Calories: 230 kcal
- Protein: 11g
- Carbohydrates: 31g
- Dietary Fiber: 4g
- Sugars: 24g
- Fat: 7g

Cooking Tips: Feel free to use any combination of fresh or frozen berries you prefer. For extra flavor, you can add a touch of lemon zest or a sprinkle of cinnamon.

Recipe 56: Mediterranean Hummus Wrap

Prep Time: 15 minutes - Number of Servings: 2

Ingredients:

For the Wrap:

- 2 wholegrain or spinach tortillas
- 1 cup hummus (storebought or homemade)
- 1 cup mixed greens (spinach, arugula, or lettuce)
- 1/2 cup cherry tomatoes, halved.
- 1/2 cup cucumber thinly sliced.
- 1/4 cup red onion thinly sliced.
- 1/4 cup Kalamata olives pitted and sliced.
- 1/4 cup crumbled feta cheese (optional)
- Fresh parsley for garnish (optional)

Cooking Instructions:

1. Lay out the tortillas on a clean surface.

2. Spread a generous layer of hummus evenly over each tortilla.

3. Divide the mixed greens, cherry tomatoes, cucumber, red onion, Kalamata olives, and crumbled feta cheese (if using) evenly between the two tortillas, placing the ingredients in the center.

4. Sprinkle with fresh parsley if desired.

5. Fold in the sides of each tortilla and then roll them up tightly, creating a wrap.

6. Slice the wraps in half diagonally, if preferred, and serve immediately.

Nutritional Values:

- Calories: 350 kcal
- Protein: 12g
- Carbohydrates: 43g
- Dietary Fiber: 9g
- Sugars: 5g
- Fat: 17g

Cooking Tips: Customize your wrap with roasted red peppers, artichoke hearts, or grilled chicken for added protein. Warm the tortillas slightly before assembling the wraps to make them easier to roll.

Recipe 57: Lemon Garlic Shrimp and Asparagus

Prep Time: 10 minutes - Cooking Time: 15 minutes - Number of Servings: 4

Ingredients:

- 1-pound large shrimp, peeled and deveined
- 1 bunch fresh asparagus, trimmed and cut into 2inch pieces.
- 3 cloves garlic, minced.
- Zest and juice of 1 lemon.
- 2 tablespoons olive oil
- Salt and pepper to taste
- Fresh parsley for garnish

Cooking Instructions:

1. Combine the shrimp, asparagus, minced garlic, lemon zest, lemon juice, olive oil, salt, and pepper in a large bowl. Toss until the ingredients are well coated.

2. Preheat a large skillet over medium-high heat. Add the shrimp and asparagus mixture to the skillet.

3. Cook for 3-4 minutes, stirring occasionally, until the shrimp turns pink and opaque.

4. Once cooked, remove from heat and garnish with fresh parsley.

5. Serve immediately as a flavorful and healthy main course.

Nutritional Values:

- Calories: 200 kcal
- Protein: 24g
- Carbohydrates: 7g
- Dietary Fiber: 3g
- Sugars: 2g
- Fat: 8g

Cooking Tips: To prevent overcooking, do not overcrowd the skillet when cooking the shrimp and asparagus. Feel free to serve this dish over cooked quinoa, brown rice, or whole wheat pasta for a heartier meal.

Recipe 58: Mixed Berry Chia Pudding

Prep Time: 10 minutes - Chilling Time: 4 hours or overnight - Number of Servings: 2

Ingredients:

- 1/4 cup chia seeds
- 1 cup unsweetened almond milk (or any milk of your choice)
- 1 tablespoon honey or maple syrup (adjust to taste)
- 1/2 teaspoon vanilla extract
- 1 cup mixed berries (strawberries, blueberries, raspberries)
- Fresh mint leaves for garnish (optional)

Cooking Instructions:

1. Combine chia seeds, almond milk, honey or maple syrup, and vanilla extract in a bowl. Stir well to mix all ingredients thoroughly.

2. Cover the bowl and refrigerate for at least 4 hours or overnight. Stir occasionally during the first hour to prevent clumping.

3. Once the chia pudding has thickened, stir it well to ensure an even consistency.

4. Layer the chia pudding with mixed berries in serving glasses or bowls.

5. Garnish with fresh mint leaves if desired.

6. Serve chilled as a delightful and nutritious dessert or breakfast.

Nutritional Values:

- Calories: 180 kcal
- Protein: 5g
- Carbohydrates: 24g
- Dietary Fiber: 11g
- Sugars: 9g
- Fat: 8g

Cooking Tips: Customize your chia pudding by adding sliced almonds, shredded coconut, or a sprinkle of cinnamon. Store a larger chia pudding in the refrigerator for quick, healthy breakfasts or snacks.

Recipe 59: Avocado Chocolate Mousse

Prep Time: 10 minutes - Chilling Time: 2 hours - Number of Servings: 4

Ingredients:

- 2 ripe avocados peeled and pitted.
- 1/4 cup unsweetened cocoa powder
- 1/4 cup honey or maple syrup (adjust to taste)
- 1/2 teaspoon vanilla extract
- Pinch of salt
- Fresh berries for garnish (optional)

Cooking Instructions:

1. Place the ripe avocados, cocoa powder, honey or maple syrup, vanilla extract, and a pinch of salt in a food processor or blender.

2. Blend until all the ingredients are well combined, smooth, and creamy.

3. Taste the mousse and adjust the sweetness if needed by adding more honey or maple syrup.

4. Spoon the chocolate avocado mousse into serving glasses or bowls.

5. Cover and refrigerate for at least 2 hours to chill and set.

6. Just before serving, garnish with fresh berries if desired.

7. Serve chilled as a guilt-free and creamy dessert.

Nutritional Values:

- Calories: 170 kcal
- Protein: 2g
- Carbohydrates: 21g
- Dietary Fiber: 6g
- Sugars: 12g
- Fat: 11g

Cooking Tips: You can use either honey or maple syrup as a sweetener, depending on your preference. Add a sprinkle of grated dark chocolate or a dollop of whipped cream for extra indulgence.

Recipe 60: Sweet Potato and Black Bean Breakfast Burrito

Prep Time: 15 minutes - Cooking Time: 20 minutes - Number of Servings: 4

Ingredients:
For the Filling:

- 2 large, sweet potatoes peeled and diced.
- 1 (15ounce) can black beans, drained and rinsed
- 1 teaspoon ground cumin
- 1/2 teaspoon chili powder
- Salt and pepper to taste
- 2 tablespoons olive oil
- 1/2 cup diced red bell pepper.
- 1/2 cup diced red onion.
- 1/4 cup chopped fresh cilantro.

For the Burritos:

- 4 wholegrain or spinach tortillas
- 4 large eggs, scrambled.
- 1/2 cup shredded cheddar cheese (optional)
- Salsa for serving (optional)

Cooking Instructions:
For the Filling:

1. Heat the olive oil over medium heat in a large skillet. Add the diced sweet potatoes and sauté for about 8-10 minutes or until tender and slightly browned.

2. Add the diced red bell pepper, red onion, ground cumin, chili powder, salt, and pepper to the skillet. Sauté for another 3-4 minutes until the vegetables are softened.

3. Stir in the black beans and cook for 2-3 minutes until heated through.

4. Remove the skillet from heat and sprinkle fresh cilantro over the filling.

Assembly:

1. Warm the tortillas in the microwave for about 20 seconds to make them pliable.

2. Add a portion of the scrambled eggs on each tortilla, followed by a scoop of the sweet potato and black bean filling.

3. If desired, sprinkle shredded cheddar cheese over the filling.

4. Fold in the sides of each tortilla and then roll them up tightly, creating a burrito.

5. Serve the breakfast burritos with salsa on the side if you like.

Nutritional Values:

- Calories: 320 kcal
- Protein: 10g
- Carbohydrates: 47g
- Dietary Fiber: 11g
- Sugars: 7g
- Fat: 11g

Chapter 10: Conclusion

As we end our journey through the "Osteoporosis Diet Cookbook, "it's important to summarize the points and highlight the importance of maintaining a bone diet for managing osteoporosis. This cookbook was created to provide nutritious recipes that prioritize bone health while satisfying your taste buds.

Main Points:

1. Calcium and Vitamin D Are Vital: It is crucial to ensure an intake of calcium and vitamin D to maintain healthy bones. Include calcium foods such as dairy products, leafy greens, and fortified options. Also, spend some time outdoors to get vitamin D from sunlight exposure.

2. Balanced Nutrition Makes a Difference: A rounded diet consisting of proteins, whole grains, fruits, vegetables, nuts, and seeds provides the necessary nutrients for maintaining bone health. Protein assists in collagen formation, while antioxidants from fruits and vegetables help protect bone cells.

3. Reduce Sodium and Caffeine Intake: Limit your consumption of high-sodium foods such as caffeinated beverages because excessive intake can result in calcium loss from bones. Choose low-sodium seasonings whenever possible. Consider opting for drinks.

4. Physical Activity Is Essential: Engaging in weight-bearing exercises and strength training improves bone density and overall bone health.

Remember to consult your healthcare provider or a fitness expert to determine the exercise routine that suits your needs.

5. Mindful Cooking and Eating: Introducing the recipes from this cookbook into your life can bring joy and flavor to managing osteoporosis. Get creative with tastes, textures, and ingredients to keep your meals interesting and nutritious.

Maintaining a Nourishing and Delightful Approach:

Remember that managing osteoporosis doesn't mean compromising on taste or enjoyment of food. In fact, you can have a bone diet that's both delicious and satisfying. By prioritizing ingredients and following the recipes, you can embark on an exciting culinary journey that benefits your bones and overall well-being.

Stay dedicated to your choices. Seek personalized guidance from your healthcare provider as you continue towards better bone health. Your efforts to nourish your body with nutrients will contribute to building and maintaining resilient bones.

We hope this cookbook has motivated you to embrace a nourishing and flavorful approach to managing osteoporosis. You have the opportunity for a fulfilling life with bones by making food choices, staying active, and maintaining a positive mindset.

Thank you for joining us on this adventure.

Here's to years of robust bone health!

Appendix: Additional Resources

In your journey toward better bone health and managing osteoporosis, it's essential to have access to reliable sources of information and support. This appendix lists websites, books, and organizations offering valuable resources for further information on osteoporosis and bone-healthy diets. These resources can help you stay informed, make informed choices, and connect with communities that promote bone health.

Websites:

1. National Osteoporosis Foundation (NOF):

Website: [www.nof.org] (https://www.nof.org/)

The NOF is a leading organization dedicated to preventing osteoporosis, promoting strong bones, and providing resources for individuals with the condition. Their website offers a wealth of information on bone health, treatment options, and nutrition.

2. The International Osteoporosis Foundation (IOF):

Website: [www.osteoporosis.foundation] (https://www.osteoporosis.foundation/)

The IOF is a global alliance committed to raising awareness of osteoporosis and promoting prevention and treatment. Their website provides extensive resources on osteoporosis research, lifestyle recommendations, and patient support.

3. MedlinePlus - Osteoporosis:

Website: [www.medlineplus.gov/osteoporosis.html)

MedlinePlus, a U.S. National Library of Medicine service, offers reliable, up-to-date information on various health topics, including osteoporosis. You'll find easy-to-understand articles, videos, and links to clinical trials.

Books:

1. "The Osteoporosis Diet: The Complete Guide to Bone Health" by Lori A. Smolin and Mary B. Grosvenor:

This comprehensive book provides valuable insights into the role of nutrition in bone health. It offers practical advice on dietary choices and recipes to support strong bones.

2. "The Myth of Osteoporosis" by Gillian Sanson:

Gillian Sanson challenges common misconceptions about osteoporosis and offers a holistic approach to managing bone health through nutrition, exercise, and lifestyle changes.

3. "The Calcium Lie II: What Your Doctor Still Doesn't Know" by Robert Thompson and Kathleen Barnes:

This book delves into the importance of calcium and magnesium balance in the body and how it affects bone health. It provides insights into dietary choices that can promote optimal bone strength.

Organizations:

1. American Bone Health:

Website: [www.americanbonehealth.org]

American Bone Health is dedicated to educating the public about bone health and osteoporosis prevention. Their website offers resources, tools, and community support.

2. Osteoporosis Canada:

Website: [www.osteoporosis.ca]

Osteoporosis Canada provides valuable information and resources for Canadians concerned about bone health. They offer educational materials, support networks, and advocacy efforts.

3. International Society for Clinical Densitometry (ISCD):

Website: [www.iscd.org]

ISCD is a global organization focused on improving bone health assessment and treatment. Their website offers educational resources and guidelines for healthcare professionals and patients.

These resources serve as valuable companions to your journey toward better bone health. Whether you seek nutritional guidance, research updates, or community support, these websites, books, and organizations help you stay informed and empowered.

While these resources provide valuable information, consulting with your healthcare provider for personalized advice and treatment options tailored to your needs is essential.

About The Author

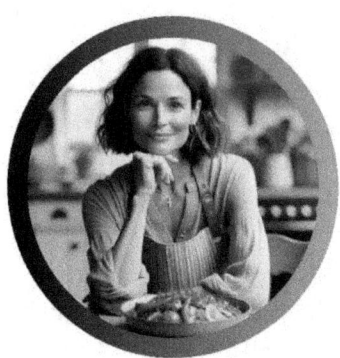

Samantha Bax, an advocate of vegan, friendly, and renal-conscious cuisine, found her true calling in the heart of a bustling city. Her journey in a professional kitchen began in her grandmother's cozy home, where she first learned the value of wholesome and nutritious eating.

When Samantha was diagnosed with diabetes in her twenties, her life turned. This pivotal moment fueled her dedication to health and wellness, ultimately leading her to become a certified nutritionist. However, when a close family member was diagnosed with kidney disease, fate had a plan for Samantha. This significant event merged her two passions for food and well-being, inspiring her to create a niche catering to diabetic and renal diets.

Course Samantha encountered challenges along the way. Balancing health requirements with flavors proved to be complex. However, she refused to compromise taste for health's sake. To overcome this hurdle, Samantha embarked on a culinary adventure where she drew inspiration from kitchens across the Mediterranean region, spice markets in Asia, and farms throughout Central America.

In "***Osteoporosis Diet Cookbook Recipes for Seniors,***" Samantha Bax masterfully combines her story with a collection of mouth-watering recipes. She firmly believes that while food is essential for survival, it should also be cherished as a celebration of life and well-being.

Osteoporosis Diet Cookbook Recipes for Seniors - Samantha Bax

In this book, she aims to offer readers a collection of recipes that cater to their needs while providing an enjoyable culinary experience.

Outside of writing and culinary experimentation, Samantha finds joy in the art of photography. She captures the essence of both cityscapes and peaceful natural landscapes. Additionally, she leads workshops and seminars where she guides individuals in making food choices that don't compromise on taste.

Other Books by Samantha Bax

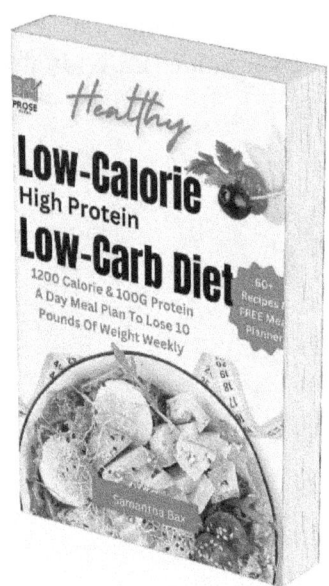 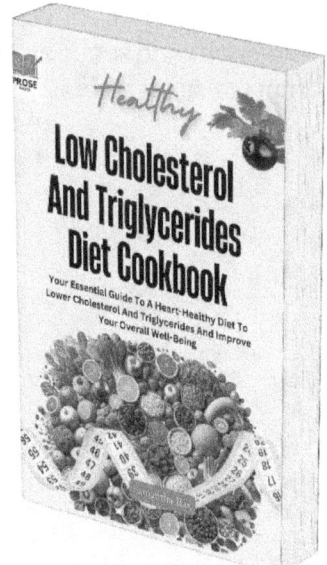 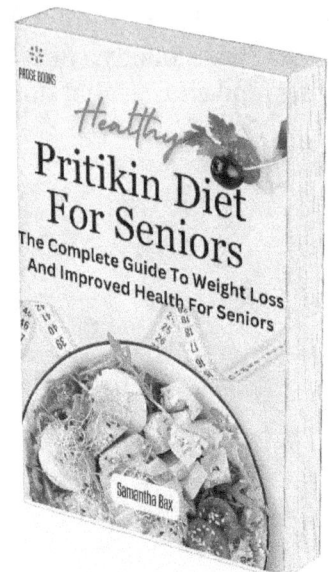

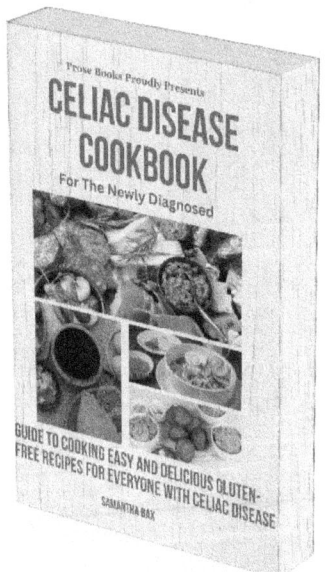 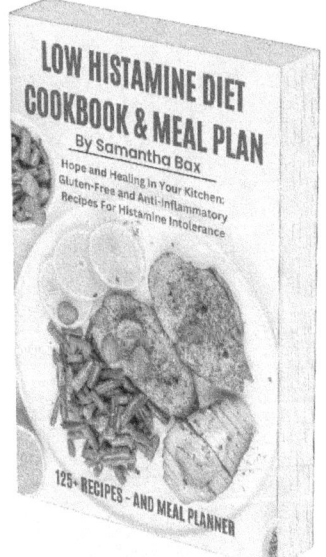 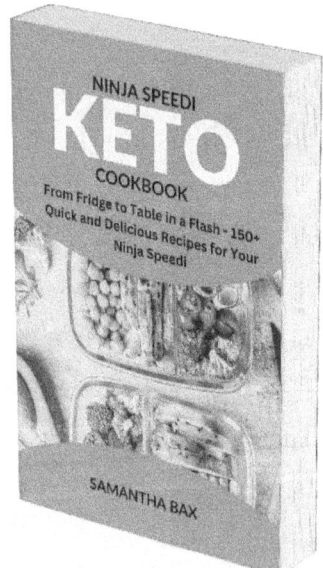

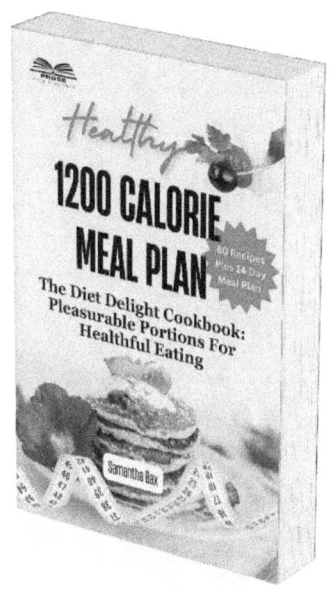
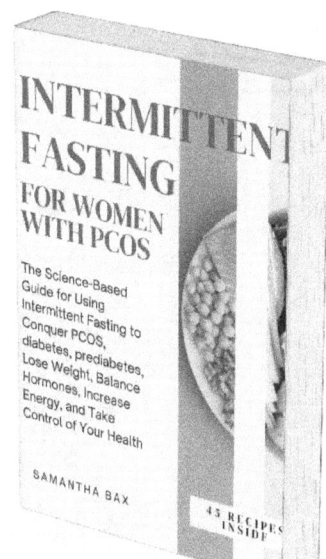
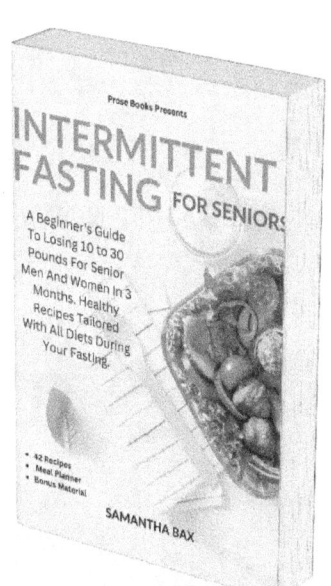
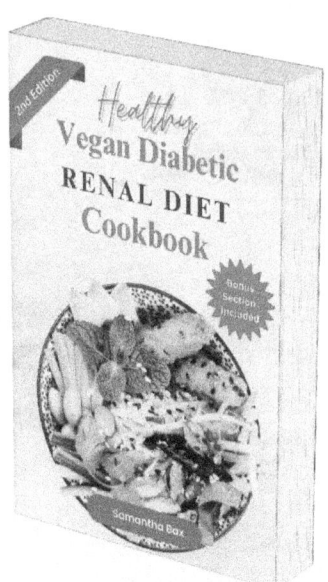
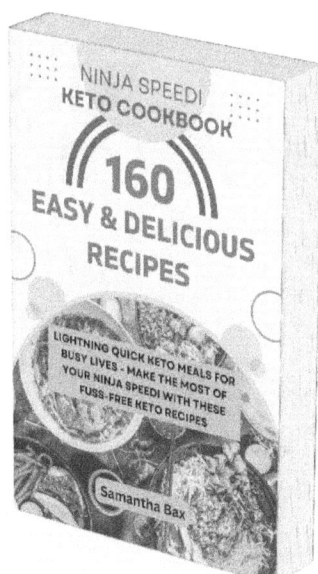
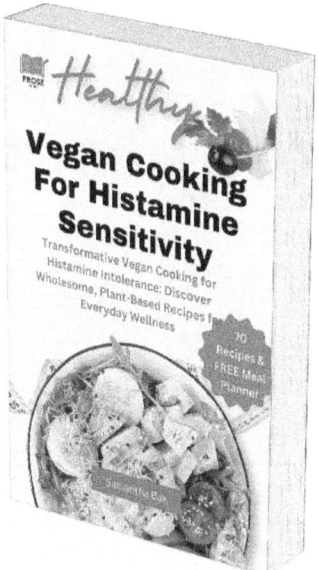

Scan the SHOP NOW code below to see all of the books and more…

https://shop.prosebooks.com

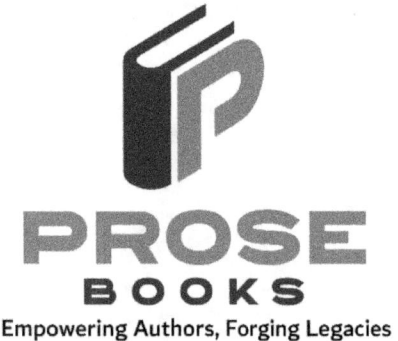

Thank You

Dear Reader,

As we approach the end of this journey, I want to express my sincere gratitude to you for embracing these recipes in your kitchen and, in turn, in your life. Your support means the world to me. It ignites my passion for sharing the goodness that food brings to our tables and our souls.

May the flavors you've explored and the nourishment you've derived from these pages inspire moments of happiness, connection, and well-being. Always remember that every meal you prepare is an expression of your imagination and thoughtfulness.

Looking forward to our escapade,

Warmest regards,

Samantha Bax

FREE Meal-Planner

As a FREE Bonus to all my readers, I invite you to go to my publisher's website at www.prosebooks.com/meal-planner and get a FREE Meal lanner to help and guide you along your journey to fitness and good health.

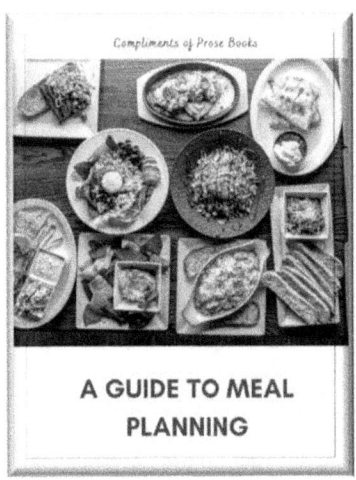

FREE Meal Planner